STORIES
FROM THE
TENTH-FLOOR
CLINIC

STORIES FROM THE TENTH-FLOOR CLINIC

A Nurse Practitioner Remembers

Marianna Crane

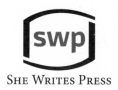

SHE WRITES PRESS

Published 2018
Printed in the United States of America
ISBN: 978-1-63152-445-5 pbk
ISBN: 978-1-63152-446-2 ebk
Library of Congress Control Number: 2018943324

For information, address:
She Writes Press
1569 Solano Ave #546
Berkeley, CA 94707

She Writes Press is a division of SparkPoint Studio, LLC.

To my patients

CONTENTS

Part Three: Playing Sheriff

Author's Note

As a new nurse practitioner in the mid-'80s, I worked in the emerging specialty of gerontology. I often grappled with how best to serve those who sought my care—poor, elderly, inner-city high-rise residents who didn't have access to adequate health services and often had to choose between food and medicine. Their multiple struggles, and my quest to provide them with the care and dignity they deserved, plagued my thoughts and dreams until I began to give voice, through writing, to our shared experiences.

To tell my story, I reread my journals, researched data, and interviewed others with whom I had worked at the time. All names have been changed to maintain confidentiality and consistency, except for those of members of my immediate family.

I hope you will enjoy getting to know this diverse group of individuals as much as I have.

PART ONE
GETTING OUT

1

Dropping In

The slap of bare feet on linoleum caught my attention before a tall, wild-haired man in boxer shorts and a sleeveless undershirt appeared in the doorway.

Dropping my pen on the desk, I shoved the chair back, ready to bolt from the room—except that he blocked the way, breathing heavily, and leaning against the door jamb. He wasn't angry. He wasn't carrying a weapon. He looked so unsteady that I probably could have pushed him over with one hand. My surging adrenalin began to subside. After all, this was a clinic.

"What can I do for you?"

"I feel lousy." He staggered into the room and plopped down on the chair next to my desk. His long, hairy legs splayed out in front of him, his arms dangled, and his head dropped to his chest. The stink of sour sweat and urine rose from him.

Just then Amanda Ringwald poked her face in the doorway, worried eyes roaming from me to the man and back. I nodded indicating that it was okay for her to go back to her desk. I had everything under control. What could she do anyway? Eighty-four years old, Mrs. R was a fixed body at the reception desk in the waiting room. She greeted patients, answered the phone, and muddled messages.

"What's your name? I asked the man.

He turned his head toward me. Bright yellow colored the sclera of his empty eyes.

"Peter Zajac." He gulped. "I live down the hall. 1002." He sucked in another deep breath before he added, "I'm sick." The scent of alcohol rode on his breath.

I recognized the name. Suddenly I recognized the man. More than once I had watched him stumble past the clinic door in a drunken stupor on the way to his apartment.

"Tell me what's wrong, Mr. Zajac."

"I feel lousy."

He didn't look critical enough to call 911, so I ran through the usual review of systems from head to toe: headache, nausea, shortness of breath, chest pain. On and on. He shook his head *no* at every question. "Do you drink?" I asked.

"Some."

"Let me check you over," I said, rolling the antique blood pressure machine across the linoleum. I listened to his heart and lungs, poked at his belly looking for pain and fluid, and checked his legs for water retention. I found his blood pressure low and his heart rate a bit fast.

Considering his jaundiced eyes and past behavior, my best guess was alcohol toxicity. He might have been hypoglycemic as well. Couldn't hurt to give him some orange juice to bring up his blood sugar.

I zipped past Mrs. R on my way to the kitchen that doubled as our supply room. Sun streamed in from the window behind her, transforming her wispy white hair into a halo. I took out a container of orange juice from the refrigerator, poured some into a plastic cup, and forced a smile in her direction before scurrying back to the exam room.

While Mr. Zajac held the cup to his lips with shaky hands, I recalled that his daughter had walked into my office a few days before. Dropping in without an appointment must run in the family. I was unpacking some items from my last job when I noticed her standing next to me. The tuning fork in my hands slipped and clanged as it hit the floor.

"Just stopped in to say hello," she said, pressing a handbag under her arm, her middle-aged face devoid of makeup. She told me her dad lived down the hall. "I'm happy that the clinic has opened on his floor. I bet you're busy with all the sick old-timers who live in this building."

"Yes," I said, when in fact we weren't. Not yet, anyway. The Senior Clinic hadn't been open long, and then only for a few hours a week— that is, until I came on board as the full-time coordinator.

Mr. Zajac's daughter chattered on. What was her point?

"Dad's killing himself with booze," she finally said, her lips quivering.

Although I had more boxes to unpack, I couldn't kick a sobbing woman out of my office. I put my arm around her shoulders, steered her to a chair, and listened to the saga of a daughter depressed over her father's self-destructive behavior.

"I can't confront your father and tell him to stop drinking. I only wish it was that easy. He needs to walk into this clinic and ask for help."

And so he did.

I eased the empty cup out of Mr. Z's hand.

"Thank you," he said, his voice stronger. He pulled back his shoulders, sitting straighter in the chair. Was it my imagination or did he seem a bit better? No doubt he had been a handsome man once. I tried picturing him in clothes.

As I mulled over what to do with him, I remembered that his daughter had told me he went to the Veterans Administration Clinic. The vise gripping the back of my neck slowly released. His daughter was right—he's killing himself with booze. I could send him back to the VA where he would be admitted to the detox unit. My last job had been over there, so I knew the ER nurses. It would be simple to arrange for an ambulance if he agreed to be hospitalized.

I pulled up a chair and sat facing him. His body odor was less repugnant—or was I adjusting to it?

"Mr. Zajac, I have something to tell you. Listen carefully."

"Yes," he said, watching my face.

"You're a sick man. We need to find out what's wrong with you so you can get better. I don't have the equipment in this clinic to help you. You should be in a hospital where they can do the tests to find out why you feel so lousy." I decided not to mention the detox unit. The hospital staff could deal with that.

"You're already a patient at the VA, right?" He bobbed his head. "I could call them and get you admitted. Is this okay with you?" I held my breath. His brow wrinkled and his jaw, covered with gray and brown stubble, began to rotate like he was chewing his cud, actions I hoped meant he was considering my suggestion.

He slowly bobbed his head again.

Hallelujah.

One last hurdle before I called the VA.

"I need to see your VA card. Please go back to your apartment and get it for me."

Standing in front of him, I bent my knees and centered myself before I offered him my hand.

"Let's see how you do on your feet." With a tug and a grunt, he

stretched his ungainly body to full height. Looming over me, he stead-
ied himself before releasing my hand.

"Okay, good to go. Get your card and come on back to the clinic."

I felt relieved as I watched Mr. Z shuffle out in his grubby underwear. I have always been ill at ease around drunkards. Occasionally,
when I was a child, a drunk would curl up on the floor in the foyer of
my apartment building in Jersey City, sleeping off a bender. I imagined
him as a dozing giant, easily startled when I juggled the doorknob,
rising from his stupor to run after me and break my bones. Luckily,
I could enter the next apartment building to get to mine through a
common backyard. Although I had avoided harm, these nameless
men had often invaded my childhood dreams.

Twenty minutes later, a door slammed and feet scuffed down the
hall. Mr. Z had managed to dress himself in a flannel shirt, rumpled
trousers, and slippers. He stumbled through the doorway and lurched
forward. His feet shuffled faster and faster, trying to stay upright. I
ran toward him but was too late. His knees hit the ground. His chest
slithered along the floor, while his arms slid out in front of him, cush-
ioning his head. A purple card bounced out of his hand.

I knelt beside him, relieved he was still breathing and that he
hadn't hit his head.

"Are you hurt?" I asked.

"No," he whispered. Cautiously, I moved his extremities. Nothing
seemed broken. I didn't try to get him up. He was safer on the floor.

As I sat back on my heels, he groaned and rolled onto his side, away
from me. His legs jackknifed to his chest. A cough rattled in his throat.
Dark, slimy liquid spewed from his mouth. I smelled the sweet musty
scent of blood. I hated that smell.

My whole body tensed. He was an alcoholic. He might burst one of
the varices—dilated blood vessels—in his esophagus that most heavy

drinkers had. What if he bled out right here? I had cared for alcoholic patients when I worked in a medical intensive care unit in the 1970s, spending many a night flushing ice water into a tube threaded down their throats to prevent the varices from bleeding. That was when I developed a deep aversion to the smell of blood.

No time to call the VA. I pushed myself up from the floor, reached for the phone on my desk and dialed 911.

"This is Marianna Crane, nurse practitioner. I run the Senior Clinic on the tenth floor in the Chicago Housing Authority building on North Noble." I took a deep breath to slow the rush of my words. "I have a patient in the office who is weak, sweaty, and has vomited blood. I need an ambulance."

Sometimes ambulances delayed coming into a neighborhood considered unsafe. While the community surrounding the building had its share of gang activity and I wouldn't walk alone at night, there were worse neighborhoods on the West Side. I hoped my credentials and the fact I was calling from a clinic would bring the ambulance quickly.

I retrieved Mr. Z's purple card from the floor. The color indicated that he was entitled to full veteran services. If his condition stabilized at the community hospital, he could be transferred to the VA.

I stepped over Mr. Z and pulled two threadbare cotton towels from the drawer underneath the exam table. I folded the first towel and tucked it under his head.

"Better?"

He grunted.

On my way to the kitchen to wet the second towel, I stopped in front of Mrs. R's desk. No other patients were in the waiting room— the living room–dining room of a converted one-bedroom apartment. I told her I had called an ambulance.

"When they buzz, just let them in."

I patted Mr. Z's mouth with the damp towel and tried to flick bits of vomitus off his chin. With the same towel I wiped up the bloody mess.

In spite of Mr. Z's noisy respirations, he looked comfortable—like the drunks of my childhood sleeping in my apartment foyer. While I didn't fear Mr. Z would rise and attack me, I did worry he might pop a blood vessel. I had left a state-of-the-art clinical set-up at the VA. If Mr. Z had shown up there, he would now be in a hospital bed, not lying here on the floor waiting for an ambulance that might not come.

But it did, within twenty minutes of my calling. Through the window I watched the paramedics lift Mr. Z into the ambulance. "Thank you, Jesus," I said under my breath as the ambulance raced out of sight.

Armed with a package of brown paper towels and a spray can of disinfectant, I did battle with Mr. Z's lingering odor. I wrote a note to his daughter telling her that her father was at Saint Elizabeth Hospital, then folded and put it, along with Mr. Z's VA card, into an envelope. On the outside I scribbled *For Mr. Zajac's Daughter,* since I didn't know her name. I taped the note to his apartment door.

Walking past the other closed apartment doors on my way back to the clinic, I wondered what surprises were holed up behind them. Who else might stumble into the clinic with a heart attack, gunshot wound, or psychotic episode? I hadn't planned on running an emergency room.

But then I had accepted the position without a thorough appraisal. Had I been that anxious to leave my old job? What in God's name kind of place was this?

2

A Difficult Decision

I n 1983, after working at the VA for almost four years, I was assigned
to recruit for a research study.

Hunkered down in my basement TV room, I'd been making phone
calls to eligible patients. From the computer files I sought men with
high blood pressure and no serious heart problems who would agree
to take one of two medications.

"Hi, I'm Marianna Crane, a nurse practitioner. I work at the VA
Hospital."

My introduction usually precipitated a deep silence on the line.
Some of the men may have been waiting for bad news I might give
them or were calculating the retribution I could take on them if they
hung up. So I hurried through my spiel.

"I'm calling to invite you to be part of a hypertension study. If you
qualify, you will get free medication and follow-up care for the next
six months."

My family knew not to disturb me while I made the phone calls. I
could hear Mom treading on the wooden floor in the kitchen above

me as she cooked dinner. Ernie was in the living room smoking his pipe and reading the *Tribune*. Two flights up, Doug had sealed himself in his bedroom and was working on his computer. Jeannine was listening to her music—or rather one song on the record player, loudly and repeatedly. Before I came down, I had asked her to close her bedroom door, but strains of "Uptown Girl" traveled though the air ducts competing with the hum of the furnace.

After deciding the noise level wasn't intrusive, I dialed the first number. I planned to return to the basement after dinner. My last call late that evening nabbed Gus.

The next morning, I drove out early into frigid January blackness to meet Gus, a policeman. He had to get to work—first shift—on time. I drove through the main gate of the VA complex, past the new hospital. The entrance to the psychiatric center was closest to my office. Even on that cold, dark morning, four men in heavy jackets stood outside under the streetlights, smoking. I turned off the engine, rolled down the window, and watched them. None paced, mumbled to himself or otherwise behaved erratically, so I got out of the car and locked the door. As I strolled toward them I could feel their eyes penetrating my thick down coat.

One of the men opened the door to let me in. His breath billowed white as he uttered, "Good morning." Once inside the hospital, I glanced over my shoulder to see if any of them were following me. I never did plan what to do if one came after me.

At the end of a prefab suite wedged along the corridor in the old building, I unlocked the private entrance to my office. Dr. Leon Logan, who ran the Geriatric Department, had given me the largest office after his. A mound of patients' charts that I hadn't finished looking over covered my desk. Most of them were thick with information because our clinic enrolled only patients over sixty-five with a long history of hospital admissions.

The VA, like other health facilities in the early 1980s, was seeing an increased number of geriatric patients. The literature suggested that interdisciplinary teams such as ours—Leon Logan (physician), Meg Brennan (social worker), and I (nurse practitioner)—that collectively took care of elderly patients could cut costs while improving their health.

I put on my government-issue drab-white lab coat, made for males, which fitted me poorly—baggy shoulders, long sleeves—and a snug skirt. I pinned on my nametag: Marianna Crane, RN, MS, GNP, the latter for Gerontological Nurse Practitioner.

My steps echoed down the dim hallway as I passed rows of empty seats. A sandy-haired, muscular man in a dark blue uniform sat stiffly in one of the chairs in a cul-de-sac off the main corridor. He smiled, showing bright white teeth, and his good looks made me wonder why the hell I had decided to specialize in geriatrics.

After we exchanged pleasantries, I gave him my canned speech. "Thank you for coming, Gus. Your participation in the study will help doctors learn which blood pressure medicine works best."

I unlocked one of the exam rooms our Geriatric Clinic used three mornings a week.

"Unbutton your shirt so I can listen to your heart and lungs, please."

Gus put his policeman's hat on the chair and began to open his shirt. I kept my eyes on the floor.

"The VA has been good to me. I'm happy to do anything I can for the other vets," he said. Most of the guys I interviewed said pretty much the same thing. The one positive aspect to the recruiting gig was meeting the vets who agreed to participate.

Gus's lungs were clear and his heart sounds were normal. There was so much pathology in my older patients that I had almost forgotten what young, healthy lungs and hearts sounded like.

I finished with Gus before the clinic officially opened. He went off to work, and I headed back to my office.

Meg Brennan shuffled about in her cozy cubicle, sandwiched between the secretary's office and the coffee room. She was a dedicated social worker who came in early or stayed late to get her job done. We had worked well together for the last three years.

"Morning, Meg."

"So how's recruitment going?" she asked, pulling off her boots.

"I enrolled another patient," I said. "Just three more to go."

Meg's long chestnut hair, porcelain skin, and short stature made her look younger than thirty-three. Without a wedding ring, she received unwanted attention from the veterans. Sometimes I did, too, even though I was eight years older and wore a wedding ring.

Just a few weeks before, Mr. Hill, a tall, lanky seventy-eight-year-old dairy farmer from southern Illinois, had come in for an evaluation of his blood pressure and COPD, a lung disease. His wife and daughter had just left the exam room. I clutched the Christmas tin with cookies Mrs. Hill had baked for my team and stepped back to let Mr. Hill leave the room before me.

"How about a Christmas kiss?" Mr. Hill grabbed me round the waist and pressed me against his potbelly. My nose smashed into the pack of Lucky Strikes in the pocket of his flannel shirt. The heavy dosing of Old Spice didn't cover the scent of tobacco exuding from in his body. I felt violated. How could Mr. Hill disrespect my professional position?

"Mr. Hill, let me go," I softly hissed, lest his family hear. Shoving the cookie tin into his gut, I broke his grip. Eyes downcast, he shuffled out of the room behind me.

Later, I wondered why I attempted to protected Mr. Hill's reputation. He had perhaps been a womanizer his whole married life. It was a good lesson for me that older men were not innocent, asexual creatures.

I was learning on the job since few formal educational opportunities to study aging existed in the late 1970s and early 1980s. Although my nametag said *Gerontological NP*, I had taken only two elective classes in geriatrics in my master's program—Chronic Disease in the Elderly I and II. Leon hadn't had any formal training. A board certification exam in geriatric medicine didn't exist. Even so, he had been hired to start the Geriatric Program.

Nursing, at least, was working on a Gerontological NP certification, but a test had yet to be developed. I had become certified by writing a case study about a patient who was one of the few still alive who had served in World War I.

As part of my job, the nursing department at the VA asked that I speak to new nursing employees about gerontology. I asked Meg to join me in conducting the monthly orientation session. Working with her would demonstrate how well other disciplines could collaborate with nurses.

I described the normal aging process and what nurses could do to deal with some peculiar problems seen in older patients, such as *sundowning*: increased mental confusion that occurs as daylight begins to fade. Common practice was to sedate the patient, usually with a drug called Haldol, and raise the side rails to keep the patient in her hospital bed all night.

"What often happens," I told the nurses, "is that the patient experiences agitation and dizziness—side-effects of Haldol—climbs over the side rails, and falls to the floor, breaking a hip."

Sometimes nurses restrained, or tied, the patient to the bed. At worst the patient might twist about, the restraints strangulating her and causing death. If not death, then an agitated, sleep-deprived patient becoming more and more confused.

"Better to lower the bed," I said. "Place a night light in the room and check the patient frequently, walking her to the bathroom as needed." But this would take up much more of the nurse's time. What would change nursing practice other than a major shift in attitude toward caring for the aging population? And that was what Meg and I strove to do in our workshop.

Meg conducted an experiential exercise. She asked the nurses to relax, close their eyes, and picture themselves in front of a mirror. Then she had them "see" themselves in progressively older stages of life—from childhood, until finally . . .

"Now you're eighty years old." Her voice was soothing and soft, pausing between each question. "What do you see? How do you feel? How are you dressed? What's important to you?"

Once I was approached by a short, Hispanic male in his late twenties.

"Don't you work at the VA?"

"Yes," I said, surprised to be asked that question in the produce section of Dominic's grocery store.

"Wait here," he commanded.

What was going on? Who the hell was this man?

He dragged over a woman his age. "This is my wife, I want her to meet you."

He turned to his wife. "Honey, this is one of the women who gave the class."

The class. What class?

"Oh, my goodness. He talks all the time about that class at the VA. The aging class. He loved it!"

Even so, Meg and I would, as a matter of course, excuse anyone who didn't want to participate in Meg's activity. Silent tears ran down attendees' cheeks as they remembered sad or painful moments. On one occasion, soon after the start of the exercise, a middle-aged woman slammed her notebook on the desk, snatched her purse and coat, and stormed out of the room.

After hearing Meg and me discuss the sessions, Leon dubbed us the *Sob Sisters.*

✳✳✳

After conducting many of these classes, Meg and I suspected that the attendees who enjoyed our presentation were ones who had had an older person in their lives and recalled pleasant memories of the relationship. Surprising to me was how many of the nurses had no experience with older folks. They were often the ones who held tight to the negative stereotypes of aging.

Meg's maternal grandmother had lived with her family when she was little, and for a time they had shared a bedroom. "I have nice memories of her and the things we did together. We were 'buds.'"

My father's father, with a thick Italian accent and a white moustache that tickled my cheek when he kissed me, warmed my own memories. Plus, I had worked in a nursing home—a well-run home with low staff turnover—for a short period of time, but long enough to savor the slow pace after being an intensive-care nurse for years before. The residents bestowed many hugs and an occasional slobbery kiss as I passed out medications on the evening shift.

I had forgotten that experience the day my academic advisor and I talked about a master's thesis. In 1979, like most of my classmates, I wanted to study women—women of child-bearing age. Why did she think she had to ask me again: "What group do you REALLY enjoy caring for?" That's when I remembered the hugs in the nursing home.

The following year I graduated as one of a handful of gerontological nurse practitioners in the Chicago area, and became the first GNP to work with Leon Logan's new Geriatric Interdisciplinary Program.

Our clinic had filled up quickly with patients and their families; they didn't miss the busy, impersonal general medical clinic. Leon had submitted a grant to the Central VA Office to study what happened to patients seen by our interdisciplinary team. Did they stay healthier longer than patients followed in the general clinics? Were they hospitalized less frequently? Were they more satisfied with their care? Did the care our patients received cost less than traditional medical care?

A couple of months earlier, Leon had called Meg and me into his office. "I have good news and bad news," he said after we sat down at the oval table in the corner of the room. "The bad news is that our grant has been denied." He forced a smile and continued. "We can't expand the clinic until we receive grant money." His bogus grin couldn't conceal the disappointment in his voice.

"But the good news is that we were invited to resubmit." Leon was a bear of a man but at that moment, he looked like a seven-year-old wishing he still believed in Santa Claus.

I felt sad at the news and for the man. The clinic and the research study had been Leon Logan's dream. Meg and I plodded out of the office.

While it wasn't inevitable that the clinic would close, how long would it take to rewrite the grant, submit it, and then wait for the decision? Even if we did get the go-ahead, it would be over a year before we could begin the study.

Since we weren't needed full-time in the Geriatric Program, the Social Work department assigned Meg to spend a couple of days a week in the Nursing Home, a new one-story structure on the grounds of the VA complex. My nursing boss, Dorothy Powell, assigned me to her hypertensive study.

Meg was lucky to be still caring for older patients and using her social work skills, while I recruited research patients, a job I disliked.

When Dorothy summoned me to discuss my progress, I had an uneasy feeling. Her office was on the second floor of the old building, a four-story structure built at the turn of the century with bricks, concrete, and drafty windows that sat directly above the Geriatric Department. A healthy philodendron sat in a purple pot on the corner of her desk. I knocked on the opened door.

"It's me, Dorothy. You wanted to talk?"

She faced the tall windows behind her desk watching the heavy snowflakes cloud the view. She turned in her chair steadying a china cup and saucer in her hands. Raising the cup to her lips, she drank slowly. Her long blond hair framed her inexpressive face. I stood until she settled the cup on the saucer and placed them both on the uncluttered desk.

"Sit down," she said. Our friendly relationship had turned dark and distant.

"I'm dissatisfied with patient recruitment. You need to enroll more subjects."

A sinking sensation of vulnerability rippled through my body. Why hadn't she let on before this? I had seen her mood descending each time we met, and had asked if there was a problem. Each time she'd said "no."

"I think you should give more of your time to recruitment—after all, nursing is paying your salary." Her voice ratcheted up to a whine, as if all her anger toward me was escaping white-hot from her core.

She was my boss. Her word carried more weight than mine. In all my twenty years of nursing, I had never been told that my performance was unsatisfactory. My reputation was now on the line. How had I missed the clues?

I didn't tell anyone, especially Meg or Leon, that I was looking for another job. While I was hoping against hope that the Geriatric Program would get funded somehow, I needed to hedge my bets. Working with Dorothy Powell was no longer an option.

3

Getting Out

One morning, Dorothy charged into Leon's office and slammed the door. I set the coffee carafe down on the counter. There was no need to tiptoe over and press my ear to the door. Their loud, angry voices filled the outer room as they argued about where I should spend my time.

I carried my coffee cup to my desk and waited out the storm. How could they meet without me? Didn't I have a say in where I would work? When Dorothy's footsteps clopped out of Leon's office, I stormed in. I stopped short when I saw him hunched over with his chin resting on both hands. He signed deeply and slid a sheet of paper across his desk.

"Sorry," he said.

I picked up the memo. It outlined my duties. I was to give more of my time to Dorothy's research project than to the clinic. Clearly, I was being pushed out of the Geriatric Program. Both Leon and Dorothy had signed their names at the bottom of the paper. A blank line awaited mine.

The next day, I handed in my resignation.

When Leon was told that he could not hire my replacement, he had no choice but to close the clinic. Just like that, the innovative program he had launched was gone.

I wanted to hate Dorothy Powell for forcing me to resign. But while I didn't much like the woman, I knew that VA administration's lack of support for Geriatrics was the real culprit. Meg's position within the Social Work department appeared secure. But how long could Leon hold on without an outpatient clinic? As for me, I began to comb the Want Ads.

∗∗∗

The three of us—Leon, Meg and I—met with each one of our patients and family, if they had any. Most took the news well, at least while they were in the examination room with us.

All these years later, however, one patient's reaction stands out. Clive Perkins had no family. He was one of our younger patients—in his early seventies. Clive was short and stocky with a gray crew cut. He kept all his appointments. I suspected he was lonely and our clinic gave him some social interaction.

After we told him our news, he sat on the exam table, stone-faced, his body frozen and his shoes neatly parked on the floor. He stared straight ahead, his eyes misting. The three of us waited for a nod, a shrug, a cuss word, anything. But before any of us broke the silence, Clive slid off the table, snatched his shoes, pulled open the door and slammed it shut behind him. He also slammed my heart. I could no longer deny the effect the closure of our clinic had on our vulnerable patients.

At the end of my last day, I sat in my office long after everyone else had left. The bookshelves were empty. On my desk sat two boxes which I had yet to move to my car, right by the exit in a no-parking zone. The VA police would surely ticket me if I didn't move it soon.

I had found another job. Only two were advertised for a Gerontological NP—one in a hospital setting and the other in a new clinic. I chose the latter. Along with autonomy to practice as an NP in a community setting, I would receive a reduction in pay. But what choice did I have? I had to get out.

The sound of footsteps interrupted my thoughts. I jumped at the shadow by the door.

"Hi," David Blankenship said. He was another patient who seemed to live at the VA. It wasn't unusual for him to show up at my office at odd hours with various requests. Not a gregarious man, Mr. Blankenship never took up much time making small talk. He had a depressed demeanor, narcissistic leanings, and was passive-aggressive, besides having multiple chronic physical ailments. I had referred him to the psychologist for his mood disorder and I, in turn, sought her counsel to help me deal with him. It didn't help that he had an eerie resemblance to Jack Nicholson in *The Shining*.

"Can I carry that for you?" he said, nodding his head towards the boxes on my desk.

"Sure."

I opened the trunk of my car and Mr. Blankenship silently placed the first box inside.

Back in my office I put on my coat and grabbed my purse while he lifted the last box off my desk, again without a word.

After he slammed the trunk, Mr. Blankenship walked toward me, his face flat and his eyes sad.

"Good luck with your new job."

"Good luck to you, too. Take care of yourself."

As I drove into the dark night, Mr. Blankenship's silhouette, like the dreams for our clinic, receded in my rear-view mirror.

PART TWO

WILD GOOSE CHASE

4

The Senior Clinic

Karen Cranston, my new boss, waited outside the entrance of the Chicago Housing Authority (CHA) twenty-story apartment building on Chicago's west side to show me the Senior Clinic for the first time. Although I had spent the last two weeks with Karen learning about the organization at the main center, a short walk away, I hadn't yet visited the clinic I was hired to manage.

I turned up my coat collar, bent into the chilly March wind, and trudged up the long concrete walkway to the front of the building. Karen held open one of the glass doors for me.

"Come on inside where it's warmer," she said after greeting me.

I squeezed past her tall frame into the foyer.

Karen was the Executive Director of the Family Health Center (FHC) that served the surrounding low-income community—mainly Hispanic families. She had achieved attention from local, as well as national, nursing circles for starting one of the first nurse-managed facilities. In her late thirties, she was five years younger than I. The fact that she hired doctors to support nurse practitioners and nurse midwives, and not the other way around, had attracted me to the job.

A grid of black buttons lined the wall to our right. Next to each button was an apartment number. Karen pressed the button of apartment 1006, which had next to it a strip of white adhesive tape with "Senior Clinic" written in black marker.

A disembodied voice asked, "Who is it?"

"It's Karen. I have Marianna Crane with me."

At the sound of the buzzer, she pushed open the door. We stepped into a long, dreary corridor. Across from us, one of two elevators waited with open doors.

"We're lucky. These elevators are so unreliable and slow. Let's just hope this one is in service," she said. Inside, the strong smell of disinfectant surrounded us. She selected the twentieth floor. The doors creaked closed.

"Before we go to the clinic, I want to take you to the community room where the luncheons and social events are held."

While I was anxious to see the clinic, Karen seemed in no hurry. Why hadn't I asked to visit the Senior Clinic before I took the job? It probably wouldn't have affected my decision since I wanted to leave the politics of the VA at any cost. I took a slow, long breath and tried to relax.

We stepped off the elevator into a cavernous room with folding tables and chairs stacked against the far end. The grimy floor-to-ceiling windows blurred a spectacular view of Chicago's skyline.

"Too bad they don't clean the windows more often," Karen said and took off her heavy coat that had concealed her pregnancy.

"God, it's hot up here," I said as slipped off my coat, too.

"That's because the CHA blasts the heat out. There are no thermostats anywhere. If you want cool, you open a window."

I followed her into a smaller room with the scent of moldy food. Gunmetal-gray cabinets hung on the wall above the grease-stained stove and double stainless-steel sink. A long counter in the center of the room was probably used as a buffet table.

"Mattie and Mary can put on quite a show," Karen said. She had already filled me in about Mattie Grady and Mary Nowak, two women who would report to me. Their title, Patient Advocates, seemed incongruent with the description of the elaborate luncheons and social events they organized. The Family Health Center absorbed the cost. While the informal gatherings sounded a bit strange for a healthcare organization, I decided to reserve judgment until I learned more.

"Let's go down and see the clinic," Karen finally said. "We chose the tenth floor rather than the first because there's less chance of break-ins," Karen said after the elevator doors closed. "You know," she added, "people searching for drugs."

I was born and raised in Jersey City and had made frequent journeys across the Hudson River into New York. I elbowed my way through crowds, mastered public transportation and savored the sights and smells of the multiracial neighborhoods. I prided myself on my city smarts. I hadn't been overly concerned about crime in this west side Chicago neighborhood, in spite of getting caught in the middle of a gang fight after I interviewed for the job. Yet this statement jarred me.

We stepped off the elevator into a long hallway with closed apartment doors on either side. Another makeshift sign, with "Senior Clinic" printed with black marker on white paper and taped on the wall next to the open door directly in front of us, signified my new work site.

We walked into the one-bedroom apartment. What would have been the living room/dining room had become the waiting room. A wrinkled, white-haired woman, ensconced behind the immense mental desk, faced the open door. Behind her, casement windows displayed another view of the Chicago skyline we had seen upstairs.

A chain of mismatched chairs lined the periphery where two stout women sat.

"Marianna, I want you to meet Mrs. Ringwald, affectionately known as Mrs. R."

Mrs. R rose from the desk and tottered over to give Karen a hug, her head reaching Karen's chest. Before returning to the desk, she nodded to me. Karen had lured Mrs. R out of retirement after many years as a volunteer at FHC. She would stay until I found a permanent replacement.

Then Karen turned toward the two women. "This is Mattie Grady and Mary Nowak." Both wore polyester pantsuits with large handbags parked on the scruffy linoleum floor next to them. They appeared to be in their sixties. Karen had told me that the residents nicknamed them the *M and M Sisters.*

Mattie put out her hand first: soft and brown with a firm grip. Her dark face creased with concentration as if measuring my worth.

Mary's fair fingers brushed mine in greeting, though she gave me a genial smile.

"Before I leave, let me show you around," Karen said. She dropped her coat onto an empty chair. I hugged mine tighter to my body and followed her to the bedroom—now an examination room.

"A retired dentist donated most of the office furniture. This exam table came from the community hospital. See, it even has stirrups."

From one of the three drawers on the side of the table, she dragged out a long steel rod with a heel rest and screwed it in place. I wondered how older women could get onto the table, much less put their legs up on the stirrups. Karen opened another drawer.

"We keep the ophthalmoscope and otoscope in here."

She handed me a heavy black leather-like case. Inside rested a handle with two antique interchangeable scopes: one to examine ear canals and the other to view the background of eyes. At the VA, a permanent ophthalmoscope and otoscope was mounted on the wall next to the blood pressure machine in each exam room. It seemed I was going back in time.

As we left the room, Karen stopped in front of the door on her left.

"This is the bathroom. It's used as a conference room in a pinch." Noting my puzzled expression, she added, "For privacy."

She flung open the door and flipped on the light. A large roach skittered behind the toilet and Karen shrugged as if to say, "What can you do?" I pictured myself balanced on the ledge of the tub, discussing patient issues with a co-worker sitting on the closed toilet seat, both of us keeping half an eye out for roaches.

A rickety gooseneck lamp tilted against an old-fashioned wooden desk that was wedged into a recess near the kitchen—the blood-draw area. On the kitchen counter, glass tubes were organized by the color of their rubber stoppers: red, lavender, blue, dark green. Each color indicated a different blood test. Paper cups held needles, again color-coded, but this time to indicate size. It had been a while since I had drawn blood, but I suspected it would be part of my job. I liked drawing blood.

I cautiously opened the nearest cabinet door, bracing for roaches to leap out. Karen noticed my hesitation.

"We have our own exterminator who comes once a month. He just chases the roaches to the next apartment," she said flatly. "So far we haven't seen mice."

I stifled a shudder.

"I'll leave you to Mattie and Mary. They'll give you the real scoop," Karen said as she slipped on her coat and tied a scarf around her head, preparing for the short walk back to the main center.

"Call me if you have any questions that these women can't answer."

Karen ran out the door before I could absorb my bleak surroundings. I had enjoyed the fact that I would be the first coordinator and could set up the clinic my way, but hadn't known what rudimentary conditions I'd have to contend with. Even so, this was the best job I had found.

What choice did I have but to take on the challenge of this clinic with its roaches, dilapidated furniture, and outdated equipment? The heels of my patent-leather shoes clicked on the floor as I walked toward Mattie and Mary. Tossing my coat over a chair, I sat next to them. I tugged the skirt of my Evan-Picone suit over my knees and clasped my hands in my lap, surprised at the dampness of my palms.

5

The Pigeon Lady

"Welcome," Mattie said in a raspy voice as I dragged my chair away from the wall so I could face the women. "I'm glad we have a full-time nurse practitioner to run the clinic." In spite of her welcome I had the uneasy feeling she was sizing me up.

"Yes," Mary said, "and now we can be open more hours."

Mrs. R sat quietly as Mattie chatted about the services she and Mary provided: paying medical bills, banking, shopping, and a variety of other chores. Her voice rose and her hands danced as she detailed the free breakfast on Friday mornings and sporadic lunches they hosted to get the word out about the clinic. When she paused for a breath, Mary leaned over and placed her hand on Mattie's arm.

"Tell Ms. Crane about the Pigeon Lady."

"Better yet, let's take her down to meet Angelika," Mattie said with a quick, gap-toothed smile.

I would have preferred to remain in the clinic, checking supplies and organizing the exam room, but I didn't want to appear rude. Besides, I wondered what a Pigeon Lady looked like. We left Mrs. R grinning at her desk.

In the hallway, Mattie pushed the elevator button. "We're going to the fourth floor." Then she glanced up and down the corridor as if the apartment doors had ears.

"Angelika Moustakas always wore a kerchief around her head and went out every morning to feed the pigeons," she told me. "The folks here in the building yelled at her to stop. They believed the pigeons carried diseases. And they didn't like the mess from pigeon droppings on the sidewalk."

Mattie watched me carefully as she spoke as if to make sure I was paying attention. "No one knew her name. That's why they called her 'The Pigeon Lady.' When they didn't see her for a few days, they spread the rumor that a homeless man killed her." She widened her eyes. "And dumped her in a trash can behind the liquor store."

She paused to allow me to absorb the details of the far-fetched story. "These old folks can really gossip. You'll see."

Mary moved closer to me and I got a whiff of Lily of the Valley. The kind of old-lady scent my mother wore. "Mattie and me went down to her apartment. We thought maybe she wasn't dead after all. Her door was open."

Mattie interrupted. "The door was closed but it wasn't locked— most of the residents here leave their doors unlocked—so we went in."

I had the impression Mattie needed to show her seniority.

"The kitchen window was wide open. A pigeon was flying around. There were a couple of pigeons on the windowsill eating bread crumbs."

One of the elevators rumbled its way upward.

"Does it always take this long to get an elevator?" I asked, breaking the tension of the story.

"We're lucky they're both running today," Mary said. "They break down often. I was stuck in one of them just last week."

The thought of getting stuck in an elevator made me anxious. A red exit sign at each end of the hallway indicated the stairways. I made a mental note to take the stairs whenever possible.

Mattie was not to be deterred from the Pigeon Lady's story. "We found Angelika lying in bed with her clothes on. She didn't talk at first. We thought she didn't understand English. Mary spoke to her in Polish. She didn't understand that, either."

"Then we thought she spoke Greek," Mary added. "So we asked the two Greek sisters who live together in Apartment 1802 to come and translate."

"They said 'no.'" Mattie squinted. "They think they're better than Angelika." She rolled her shoulders as if to shake off her anger. "But then Angelika finally started to feel better and began to talk in broken English."

"How's she doing now?" I asked.

"Better," Mattie said. "But at first she looked so sick that we asked Dr. Sanchez to come over and examine her. He said she wasn't eating— that she was malnourished. And you know what he did?"

I shrugged.

"He found a can of soup in one of the cabinets. Heated it up and fed it to her."

Both women radiated rapturous expressions. I forced a smile. My lord, a doctor heats up a can of soup and he's suddenly a god. I didn't dislike Antonio Sanchez. A family practitioner, he was good-looking and very popular with the Mexican patients. And until Ingrid Braun returned from her month-long China vacation, he was my collaborating physician. I had had a chance to work with Ingrid during my orientation at the main center and felt comfortable with her.

I traced my feelings of indignation for male doctors back to my nursing school days in the 1960s. The nuns drilled into my all-women class that we had to stand when a doctor (always a man) entered the room, give up our seat if we were seated, and never question the physician's authority. After twenty-plus years, I still resented male physicians. Even those as nice as Antonio Sanchez.

Finally the elevator came. Once the doors closed, Mattie again whispered as if we could be overheard.

"When me and Mary cleaned up the apartment, we found four hundred dollars in cash and a few checks stashed away under the mattress."

"Wow, that's a heck of a lot of money. What did you do with it?"

"It's locked up in a box in the clinic. We use the money to buy food for Angelika."

The whole Pigeon Lady thing didn't sound like something the clinic should get involved in. Storing large amounts of money was asking for a break-in.

"Oh yes, and we found a dead pigeon in a shoebox in the closet, too," Mary said.

Just the thought of finding that dead bird made me shiver.

A creepy silence shrouded the fourth floor. The air became cooler as we approached the corner apartment. Mattie knocked once, then pushed the door open.

"Angelika," she yelled into the room. "We brought you a visitor."

Stark white glared from the refrigerator, stove, and sink with a bit of color from a yellow flowered dishtowel hanging on the oven door handle. Dark streaks stained the walls. Bird droppings? A cool breeze seeped in from an open window. I scanned the room for pigeons. Flying birds in close quarters terrified me.

A pale woman sat on one of two chairs at the kitchen table. A frayed shawl covered her shoulders. Gray hair poked out of the red bandana wrapped around her head.

Mary glided over to her, patted her arm and told her my name.

Angelika muttered a "ha-lo." Her pasty skin made me wonder if she might be anemic.

Mattie raised the open window even more and dusted the breadcrumbs off the ledge with her fingers, then slammed the window shut.

"Angelika insists on feeding the pigeons," she barked. "If she had her way all the windows would be wide open." She scowled at Angelika like a mother at a mischievous child.

Mary pulled a bottle of milk out of the refrigerator, poured some into a cup, and placed the cup in front of Angelika. She nudged her shoulder. "Drink."

I watched the two women fuss over Angelika, each showing concern in her own way. I reminded myself that this was my first day. Certainly it was too soon to judge Mattie and Mary's behavior. However, I had to wonder what all this fussing had to do with running a clinic.

6

Home

On my drive home through heavy traffic, the dreary clinic, rickety elevators, antique equipment, and outdated furniture, along with the fussy attention showered on the Pigeon Lady, crowded my thoughts. I reminded myself of the positive aspects of the job: I was in charge of the clinic. I could run things my way. Patients would call and make an appointment to see me. I would take care of them, calling Ingrid Braun only if I needed her help. Best of all, I was out of the rigid hospital setting that limited what I could do for my patients.

As I turned into the alley behind the house, I snatched the remote from the sun visor. The garage door screeched open. I eased my beat-up, red Datsun into its narrow space, avoiding the garden tools hanging on the wall. Shafts of light pierced the gaps in the clapboard. The car stopped inches away from my son's bike leaning against the back of the garage.

Under a darkening sky, I trudged over the concrete path that wound past the mulberry tree. Every spring the bumpy berries dropped, clung to the soles of our shoes, and stained our rugs. I hated to cut the tree down, though, because it hid the backside of the dilapidated garage.

Mittens, the runt of the litter, bounded toward me and flopped on her back, blocking my way. I bent down, dropping my purse on the ground and rubbed her belly. She flipped back and forth, purring as loudly as a broken muffler. I stroked her until my legs ached and my mind had released all the images of the Senior Clinic into the cool air.

Mittens scampered up the steps and waited for me to open the side door into the kitchen. Just inside, warmth and an aroma of sizzling onions surrounded me.

"Something smells good," I said to my mother who stood at the stove. I hoped not to startle her. Her hearing was poor and she refused to be fitted for a hearing aid. Instead she complained that we all mumbled.

Mom turned from the stove, a bib apron covering her housedress. Once a tall, freckled, strawberry blond, over time she had shrunk, thickened, and faded.

"I'm making meat loaf with onion gravy, mashed potatoes, and green beans." She announced the dinner menu as if she were proclaiming mealtime as a national event.

"And, oh yes, home-made applesauce." She was a good cook but not too innovative. Okay with me since I disliked kitchen duty and Ernie and the kids loved her cooking.

"Hi, Mom," Jeannine called to me from the dining room.

"Yum," I said into my mother's right ear, rubbing her shoulder as I passed her.

Dim light filtered though the French doors. Books and papers cluttered the heavy cherry table that dominated the dining room and clashed with our modern taste. Ernie and I had bought it from a family that lived above us in married-student housing. The table was a reminder of our poor days when Ernie had left his first career, pharmacy, to earn a master's degree in Hospital Administration at the University of Chicago. My salary from a part-time nursing job paid the rent and grocery bills but not much else.

"Hi, Mom Crane," said Annie Ling, sitting at the other end of the table. Her straight black hair was pulled back into a tight ponytail. The two thirteen-year-olds were surprisingly motivated to get their homework done right after school.

"How was your day?" Jeannine asked, braces flashing through her grin.

"Just fine."

I doled out information about my nursing jobs in small sound-bites. I'd been doing this for so long no one seemed to notice. When I came home I wanted to forget work. I also knew my kids and husband would worry if they knew the daily risks of my job. Did they really need to know my new clinic was on the tenth floor to discourage drug seekers?

"Can Annie eat supper with us?" Jeannine asked.

"Sure," I said, knowing my mother wouldn't like that.

I hung up my jacket on the coat rack in the foyer. The large living room to my left probably had been two rooms: a sitting room and a music room. In an attempt to modernize the home, a former owner had ripped out the pocket doors that would have divided them. Still, Ernie and I fell in love with the old Victorian-style house; it had been built in 1908, making it one year younger than my mother.

At the top of the stairs, I passed Doug's empty room. Lately, he had been going to a friend's house after school. The master bedroom, at the other end of the hall, had its own bathroom—the first time Ernie and I didn't have to share one with our children. In one corner was a desk that we did share. A small-screen computer had replaced the electric typewriter I had used in the summer heat, just three years earlier, to pound out my Master's thesis while my glasses floated on a stream of sweat down the bridge of my nose. The house had no central air. I can still picture Doug and Jeannine, then thirteen and eleven, standing silently beside my chair waiting for me to take a typing break before they dared speak. One error and I had to retype the whole damn page. I had flunked typing in high school.

After changing into a pair of jeans, I went downstairs.

During dinner, Jeannine and Doug teased each other while Annie giggled, her attention more on Doug than on food. Doug seemed unaware that he attracted interest from his sister's friends. Mom's clenched lips appeared evident only to me. While Ernie concentrated on the meatloaf, my gut knotted watching Mom glare at Annie. I didn't rehash the scene until Ernie and I were getting ready for bed.

"She's getting worse. She acts like Jeannine and Doug's friends are stealing our food." I sat at the side of the bed slipping off my jeans. "Soon they won't want to come to our house at all after school. Doug is at his friend's house more often than he comes home."

Ernie, sitting next to me, unlaced his shoes, and listened. He never said anything to disparage Mom. He left that to me. He probably felt bad hearing my complaints since he had been the one to suggest she leave her large home in Jersey City and come to the Midwest to live with me, her only child, and her grandchildren.

At first I had resisted, remembering her moody personality. Always one to overreact to the slightest real or imagined criticism, my mother had punished my father and me with days of icy silence. I spent my childhood tiptoeing around my mother's moods. She enjoyed being the center of attention, and felt her opinions were always correct. Out of earshot of the kids, Ernie and I dubbed her "The Queen."

However, Mom was growing older, the long car trips to visit her had became tedious, and the love she shared with her grandchildren had little resemblance to what I remembered sharing with her as a child, so I finally asked her to live with us. Jeannine was seven and Doug nine when Mom came to Chicago, devoting herself to their happiness. But once they hit the teen years and wanted to spend more time with their friends and less with Nana, Mom's angry, hypersensitive personality began to resurface. At first she criticized them: *Doug's room is a mess. Jeannine plays her music too loud. They aren't eating enough.* Recently, she had turned her attention to their friends.

Siding with the kids against Mom only added to my stockpile of guilt. Without her, I wouldn't have been able to go back to school full-time for a master's degree in Public Health Nursing, nor could Ernie and I have traveled to Europe; I certainly wouldn't be working full-time.

After I turned off the light, I lay awake, knowing that a confrontation with Mom was inevitable. A familiar gut pain I had had as a child returned and warded off sleep.

7

Interfering

Sam Levy, the building manager, strolled into the exam room wearing his polyester pants and knit shirt, and plopped himself in the chair by my desk.

"I brought ya some business," he said, giving me a crooked smile topped with a salt-and-pepper mustache.

Now what? This was the third time since I started working, over a month before, that Sam had walked into my office asking a favor.

"Thelma slipped and fell outside my office just a few minutes ago and banged her arm up."

I closed the patient chart I was working on. Sam picked up a pencil and tapped the eraser on the desk while he continued in his used-car-salesman's voice that didn't give me a chance to break in.

"Luther was mopping. Guess Thelma didn't see the wet floor sign. Could ya look at her? She's in the waiting room."

Before I could ask who Thelma was, he flipped the pencil—it landed just where he had found it—and shot out of the room.

Soon after I started, Mattie had taken me to Sam's office, behind the empty reception desk on the first floor. He had been manager of the high-rise for the past twenty years.

"Most don't last that long," she said as we entered. A huge desk dwarfed a compact man hunched over an array of papers.

After Mattie introduced us, he leapt from his chair, jogged around the desk, and gripped my hand.

"Glad ta meet ya. We're gonna work well together." Then he added, "I'm sure happy to have the clinic in my building."

Sam was paid by the Chicago Housing Authority to manage the twenty-story building. My tenth-floor clinic was rented from the CHA. I didn't report to Sam, but he acted as if I did.

Sam came back into the exam room, cupping the elbow of a scrawny woman with tufts of white hair jutting from her head. He eased her down in the chair he had just vacated.

"Ms. Crane will take good care of you, honey. See ya later," Sam said, and darted out the door.

What had happened? Sam using me to placate the injured? Was I a foil in a potential liability claim? I hadn't agreed to see this woman but there she was sitting beside my desk like a scared five-year-old with chin hairs.

I introduced myself. "Did you know we opened this clinic here in the building?"

Thelma's mouth managed a wisp of a smile.

"I'm Thelma Scruggs."

So fragile. I softened my voice. "Ms. Scruggs, Mr. Levy asked me to look at your arm. Is that all right with you?" Who was I, after all, to assume Thelma wanted to be seen?

"Sure," she mumbled.

Thelma's skin was paper-thin so it wasn't any surprise she had an abrasion. The bleeding had stopped and the wound wasn't deep.

Nothing seemed broken. After questioning her, listening to her lungs and heart, and taking her blood pressure, I believed that she had indeed fallen on the wet floor, not passed out from a mild stroke or a heart irregularity.

I washed the wound, smeared on antibacterial ointment, and covered it with a non-stick pad. I was wrapping an ace bandage around the dressing, avoiding the use of adhesive tape that might further damage her thin skin, when Sam slipped back into the room.

"How is she?" he said to me, ignoring Thelma.

"She's fine. Just a tear in the skin," I said, my back stiffening.

I turned to Thelma. "Ms. Scruggs, why don't you drop in tomorrow and I'll change the dressing." I wanted to see her again in case I had missed something.

"Come on, honey, I'll walk ya back to your apartment." Sam took Thelma by her good arm and steered her out the door.

"Thanks," he said over his shoulder.

Later in the week, I met Sam by the elevators. I told him Thelma never came back.

"I'll see how she's doing," he said.

Within the hour, he phoned me.

"I went to check on Thelma. Oh lord, what a place. Could ya look in on her? Apartment 1607." I could imagine his mustache twitching.

"Is she okay?" I asked.

"Yeah. Yeah," he said impatiently. "Go. Get back to me. Thanks."

He hung up before I could refuse.

There he went again, ordering me around. But I was too curious not to go. I decided to take Mattie with me. Better for two people to make house calls, especially when I wasn't sure what I'd find. Plus, like so many of the residents, Thelma Scruggs didn't have a phone so we had to show up unannounced. Who knew what troubled Sam?

Mattie didn't recognize Thelma's name.

"Maybe I'll know her when I see her," she said.

I positioned myself in clear sight of the peephole and knocked on Thelma's door. Mattie stood beside me, standing stiffly in anticipation of what we might find. We waited. I knocked again. I knocked a third time. Just as we were about to turn around and go back to the clinic, Thelma opened the door a crack. Her vacant expression made me reintroduce myself.

"I had hoped that you would come back to the clinic so I could check your arm."

Her expression didn't change, so I charged ahead.

"This is Mattie Grady, who works with me," I said. "Can we come in? I'd like to make sure your arm is healing okay."

Thelma opened the door wider. She was more disheveled than I remembered. A stained blouse and baggy brown slacks hung on her rail-thin body. One step into the apartment and I knew what had bothered Sam: newspapers and magazines stood in towering stacks on the floor, and on every available surface in the living room. I glanced at the front page of the *Chicago Tribune* on the heap nearest me—1979, five years before.

Mattie gasped, "Oh my God." I elbowed her, but it was too late.

Thelma's brow wrinkled and she bit her lower lip.

"Excuse the mess, but I didn't get a chance to clean up today."

I wondered if the rest of the place was as cluttered.

"Let's go to the kitchen where the light is better so I can examine your arm."

As Mattie and I filed behind Thelma through the mountains of paper, magazines, and boxes, I caught sight of a card with bright balloons. I picked it up. "Happy Birthday to Aunt Thelma. Love, Josh and Andy." No envelope to see where Josh and Andy lived. The date written inside was a couple of months ago. So she had family. I placed the card back where I found it.

White dust covered the stove and counters in the kitchen. A musty smell tickled my throat. I swallowed hard, trying not to cough. I watched Mattie scan the room. This time she kept silent.

"Do you do any cooking for yourself?"

"Why, yes. All the time."

Thelma twisted the bottom of her blouse with both hands. Watching the pained expression on her face, I wished I hadn't asked such a dumb question. Did the CHA have strict rules about how a resident kept her apartment? Stacks of paper might be a fire hazard and grounds for eviction. Sadness swept over me. I didn't have a good feeling about Thelma. How long before she would fall between the piles of trash, not to be found until the rancid odor from her decomposing body seeped into the hallway?

"May I see your arm, Ms. Scruggs?"

"Sure," she said and extended her left arm. The dressing I had put on was gone. Only a slight red mark on her skin remained. Another bandage wasn't needed.

"Looks fine," I said. "It's healing nicely."

I smiled and kept my hand on her arm.

"Come down to the clinic if you have any problems, or just stop in if you want me to take your blood pressure and weigh you."

Mattie edged in front of me.

"Did ya know we have breakfast every Friday?" she said. "Down in the community room on the first floor. Starts at eight in the morning. Stop in. It's free."

"Why, how nice," Thelma said with the barest of smiles.

"I never saw such a place," Mattie said when we were alone in the elevator.

"Me, either."

I didn't know anything about compulsive hoarding, an affliction not commonly recognized at the time. I would've called her a *pack rat*. It wasn't until I visited more apartments stuffed with papers, magazines, clothes, rotting food, and other debris that I began to recognize a pattern.

Sam phoned later. "Well, what do ya think?"

"Sam, I don't know. Her apartment's a mess, but I can't say she's not taking care of herself. Maybe her family is aware she's slipping? What are you going to do?"

"Can you check up on her? If her place gets worse, let me know?"

This time I was ready. I'd be damned if I would jump every time Sam had a problem with one of the residents. It was his job, after all, to promote the safety of the people who lived in the building. Sam probably had the address of Thelma's next of kin. He could contact someone from the family to monitor her. And he had the key to each apartment. If he was so worried, he could open an apartment door and peer inside. Or send Luther, the janitor. Sam was not going to pawn Thelma off on me.

"No, Sam. I have no reason to go back to see Ms. Scruggs. I've already told her she can come to the clinic if she wants."

I hung up the phone with a bit of remorse. What did Sam think I could do, anyway? Barge into Thelma's world and take over—not unlike Mattie and Mary? They cleaned, shopped, and organized Angelika's meals and her life. The fact that the clinic operated out of one of the apartments in the senior high-rise allowed for greater access to our patients than a freestanding neighborhood facility and made it easier to help—or to interfere. I had yet to decide where I should and could draw the line between the two.

The sound of heavy rain drew me to the window. The sky had darkened and torrents of water slammed onto the sidewalks, surged along the streets like river rapids, and swirled down into the sewers.

8

Ms. Henry and Delilah

"I ain't got no birf' certificate. My kin'r all gone," Gladys Henry told me from her wheelchair parked next to my desk. The young woman who had pushed her into the exam room went to take a seat by the door.

"The best I can figure, I'm ninety years old or thereabouts," Ms. Henry said in a strong, even voice. I had learned never to guess the age of older black women with smooth, dark skin like Ms. Henry's.

A new patient, Ms. Henry had the last appointment that Tuesday. Besides her, I had three more new patients scheduled during the week. Residents from the building and some from the neighborhood, including one of the nuns from St. Boniface Catholic Church across the street, were calling to make an appointment to see me and I was delighted.

Patients already enrolled in the clinic had been coming to visit Veronica "Ronnie" Lewis. Ronnie, a family nurse practitioner, volunteered to see patients at the Senior Clinic when it first opened until a full-time coordinator, me, was found. I worried at first that Ronnie's patients would be unhappy to switch to a new NP. But Ronnie did a fine job of promoting me, maybe because she was anxious to get back to the main center.

"I don't like it when there are no doctors here except Ingrid who only comes on Monday afternoon," Ronnie had told me.

But that was exactly what excited me to take the job in the first place. I wanted to see patients on my own. Make my own diagnoses and develop a plan of care, prescribe medication if needed. I didn't discount having Ingrid a phone call away. In her absence, the other doctors at the main center would cover for her. I wasn't a doctor, after all, but I trusted that I would know when I had a situation beyond my scope of practice. Most of the older patients I cared for had chronic health issues or needed education to stay independent for as long as they could—all well within a nurse practitioner's domain.

***

"What brings you here today?" I asked Ms. Henry.

"My toe swelled. Started yesterday. Hurts so much, I can't walk on it."

Her shoeless right foot lay on a folded kitchen towel placed on the footrest—a queen's crown displayed on a silk pillow.

"Let's see your other foot," I said. "It's good to examine both sides of the body, or in this case, both feet, to see if there are any differences."

The young woman leapt from the chair and bent to remove Ms. Henry's shoe. In comparison, the right foot was swollen, and the skin looked darker. Probably because it was red. It was hard to tell redness in patients with dark skin. I leaned over and touched the cool skin of the left foot with the back of my hand. When I touched the right one it felt warm, and Ms. Henry flinched. Her foot had all the signs of inflammation: red, warm, swollen, and painful to touch. Plus she had some loss of function since she couldn't walk on it.

"Have you had this before, Ms. Henry?"

"Yep."

"When was that?"

"About this time last year."

"What did you do for it?"

"I went over to the emergency room before y'all had this-here clinic in the building. Delilah there took me in a taxi. Right, Delilah?"

Delilah nodded.

"What did they do?"

"They gave me medicine."

"Did it help?"

"Sure did."

I didn't think Ms. Henry would remember, but I asked anyway.

"Do you know the name of the medicine they gave you?"

Delilah stood, pulled a bottle out of her dress pocket, trotted over, and placed it on my desk.

I was pleasantly surprised. "Thank you, Delilah."

The label said *indomycin*. It fit the puzzle. Gout.

"Did you have any bad reactions to this medicine?"

"Nope."

"Good, because I have this drug in the clinic."

I opened one of the kitchen cabinets containing the FHC stock of commonly prescribed drugs. I counted out a week's worth of indomycin from the large jar, poured the pills into a small plastic bottle, wrote the name and dose of the drug on a label, and attached the label to the bottle.

I didn't have to use the blank scripts Antonio Sanchez had pre-signed. Though the FHC promoted nurse practitioners' independent practice, the State of Illinois didn't allow us to prescribe medications. There was a way around this hurdle since all the doctors Karen hired agreed to sign blank scripts for the NPs and midwives to use.

My first week on the job, I had asked Sanchez for ten prescriptions thinking that they might last me a couple of weeks since we had a good supply of stock drugs. He had flipped the sheets of the prescription pad, one at a time, and scribbled his name, leaving the date blank.

"I'm going to number each one and, if you would, please write down the drug, dose and name of the patient on a separate sheet of paper," Sanchez said.

It wasn't an unreasonable request. He and I had just started to work together. Why would he trust me to use the signed scripts appropriately until he saw evidence I had good judgment in giving out medications? He was, after all, breaking the law.

We both knew that prohibiting NPs from prescribing medication was the medical profession's way to limit competition rather than a way to protect the patients. That's why NPs could legally prescribe when they worked in underserved areas—communities where doctors had no incentive to set up their practices. Sanchez wasn't doing me any favors, he was ensuring that our patients received the same care, and maybe better, than those who stepped into medical offices on upscale Michigan Avenue.

***

"Oh, bless yo' heart," Ms. Henry said when she learned she didn't have to pay for the pills.

I grabbed my notebook and wrote my instructions: how to take the pills, side effects of the medication, and under what circumstances she should call me—or send Delilah down to the clinic since Ms. Henry didn't have a phone. I gave the top sheet to Ms. Henry, and pasted the carbon copy in the chart.

"Can you read my writing, Ms. Henry?" Mattie had told me some of the folks in the apartment building couldn't read.

"No, I never learnt how."

Ms. Henry passed the note off to Delilah. I was relieved she didn't appear offended by my question.

Delilah seemed to be in her late teens or early twenties. She read my note back to me slowly but accurately.

"Any questions?" I asked.

"No, ma'am."

"I'll save you a visit to the clinic. Next week I'll stop up to your apartment to see how you are doing."

Even though my experience in gerontology was limited, I believed home visits were invaluable. How else would I learn how my patients managed at home? I wanted to see for myself if they stored their medications properly. If they had a stool by their chair so they could keep their legs elevated as I had prescribed. If their home was clean, uncluttered, had good lighting, was in a safe neighborhood. Even Leon Logan back at the VA had authorized a couple of home visits.

Ms. Henry's visit played out the scenario I envisioned for myself in the Senior Clinic. She came to see me for a health problem that I diagnosed and treated, with her agreement and cooperation. I would feel gratification if her problem was resolved and she felt better.

In the meantime, Mattie and Mary, Sam Levy, and even Mrs. R continued to involve me in issues they found among the seniors that didn't necessitate health care. Issues I didn't choose to tackle.

Maybe I should have been flattered that they had faith in my ability to deal with the array of situations. But I didn't.

9

Wild Goose Chase

After Ms. Henry and Delilah left, Mrs. R handed me a sheet of paper: Ophelia, Apartment 507.

"I told her you'll be down to see her after you were done with your patient. She's sick."

Here we go again. I was annoyed to be sent on these errands. They often turned out to be wild goose chases. Mrs. R rarely got the facts straight. In spite of my frustration, however, I did have the good sense to recognize that visiting Ophelia would be good public relations even if it was an inconvenience.

I knocked on the door of Apartment 507. In case Ophelia couldn't hear well, I rapped again, louder. Deciding not to try the doorknob, I knocked again. Sometimes my pounding brought another resident out of her apartment to see what was going on. No one appeared.

Leaning closer to the door, I listened. Was anyone walking around? Breathing loudly? Moaning with pain? I didn't view another eyeball looking at me through the peephole or glimpse shadows gliding under the door.

Another wasted effort? Or was Ophelia dead on the bathroom floor? Or did Mrs. R bungle the message again? A retired school-teacher, she had penmanship better than mine but when taking messages she had the accuracy of a second-grader. I hoped to get the okay soon to hire a full-time, paid receptionist.

I stood in front of Mrs. R panting from walking up five flights of stairs.

"Mrs. R, there was no answer at Ophelia's apartment. Are you sure she lives at 507?"

I tried to keep my voice even.

She pondered my question and then said, "Let me see."

She rummaged through the clutter on her desk while I shifted from foot to foot. Scattering the stacks about, she finally pulled out a slip of paper.

"Oh, yes, here it is," she said in her wobbly, old-lady voice. "Oh, Ophelia lives on the seventh floor, 705. Goodness me."

"Do you have a phone number, Mrs. R?"

I clenched and unclenched my fists inside the pockets of my lab coat as she searched again for what she had in hand a second ago. Picking up the scrap of paper on top of a pile of patients' charts, she studied it.

"Yes, here is her number."

"I think I'll call her before going down to the seventh floor."

I snatched the phone number from her hand and marched into the exam room, resisting the urge to slam the door behind me.

A high-pitched voice answered the phone. *Damn, I don't even have her last name.*

"Ophelia? This is Marianna Crane, the nurse practitioner from the clinic. I'm told you're not feeling well."

"On no, dear. I feel fine."

"Then why did you call the clinic?"

"I just wanted to get meals-on-wheels, dear. My next-door neighbor, Harriet, gets meals-on-wheels and she was telling me about it. I would love to have someone deliver a hot lunch to my apartment every day. Don't you think that would be a good idea? I cooked when my husband Ben was alive, bless his soul, but now that there's just me . . ."

"Good idea," I told her, having no patience for Ophelia's life history.

"I'll have one of our workers, Mrs. Grady, come down and help you arrange to have meals-on-wheels delivered to your apartment."

"Thank you, dear. What did you say your name was again?"

After I hung up, I felt guilty for being so abrupt. Ophelia might tell her friends about the curt nurse practitioner that worked in the clinic. But then maybe she was so grateful for the return phone call that she didn't notice my rudeness. What kind of geriatric specialist was I not to tolerate these old folks? And more frustrating was that I could not predict when a wild goose chase would turn out to be a real emergency.

In the meantime, I ran up and down the stairs grumbling to myself.

10

B. J., The Canary

braced myself on Monday mornings, waiting for the flurry of after-the-weekend phone calls and walk-ins. But that particular morning, it wasn't a patient but Ronnie, the NP who had served as coordinator before I came, who walked into my office. Wearing a flowing skirt and Birkenstock sandals, Ronnie carried a birdcage. Setting the cage on my desk, she pulled off the cover to reveal a yellow bird pecking at a tiny mirror anchored to the side of the cage.

"Say hello to B. J.," she said.

"What in heaven's name are you doing with a canary?"

"Juanita had heard about Angelika. 'I bet she misses her pigeons,' she said and offered to let Angelika borrow B. J. Maybe he'll help her get better."

Why wasn't I surprised to hear that the story of the Pigeon Lady had circulated among the staff at the Family Health Center?

I had all but forgotten about Angelika after Mattie and Mary had taken me to meet her. Mattie and Mary had solicited Ronnie's help when they first found Angelika, and she continued to walk from the main clinic to visit Angelika once a week. Since the clinic was quiet at that moment, I agreed to accompany Ronnie as she carried B. J. down to Angelika's apartment.

I followed behind as Ronnie edged her way down the narrow, dank stairwell, gathering her skirt with one hand, and holding the birdcage with the other. The cage swayed widely as she concentrated on her step.

Bang! The cage slammed against the wall. Bouncing down the stairs, the cage lost its cover. Then the door swung open and B. J. zoomed past my head.

Our shrieks echoed loudly around us. After the vibrations died down, we stood motionless listening for one of the residents to open a door to the stairwell and ask what was going on.

No one did.

Ronnie picked up the cover, then righted the cage, and set it on a stair with the door open.

"We have to get him back. Juanita will never forgive me for losing her bird."

"I don't see him anywhere." I said, feeling a bit dizzy as I stretched out over the rail and glanced upward, searching for a yellow blob. My palms began to sweat in anticipation of fluttering wings.

We both stood motionless, waiting. Would B. J. come back to us or would we have to leave him in the stairwell to die of thirst? How long should we wait? Before I voiced my concern to Ronnie, a breeze brushed my cheek. It was B. J. as he flew past me. He circled around Ronnie's head. He alighted at the entrance to the cage. Ronnie quickly shoved him inside and slammed the door.

"Thank goodness," she said, and pushed a strand of blond hair off her forehead.

"I'm glad he likes his cage," I said, relieved that we didn't have to spend more time waiting for him to show.

Draping the cover over the cage, Ronnie gripped the cage tightly, held it above her head, and paraded once more down the stairs.

Just as before, Angelika sat at the kitchen table. This time she wore a blue bandana. Expressionless, she was traveling somewhere in her own head.

"Here's B. J. Remember I told you I would bring him?" Ronnie said. When Ronnie planted the cage on the table and pulled off the cover, Angelika came to life, and pressed her face closer to watch B. J.

B. J., as if aware he was on display, began to warble as the short hairs on his neck fluttered in and out. Behind Angelika, Mattie turned from the sink, wiping her wet hands on her apron. As she glanced at me, her eyebrows rose in a quizzical expression as if wondering why I had shown up, since I hadn't displayed any interest in Angelika.

"What a cute canary!" Mary said, sitting on the only other chair with her hands wrapped around a cup of coffee.

A half-slice of uneaten toast sat on a plate in front of her. Two more empty plates and coffee cups on the table indicated a communal meal. I worked that observation over in my head before I concluded that Mattie and Mary provided companionship for an isolated, lonely woman. And B. J.'s presence was therapeutic, too.

As the women fussed over B. J., I thought of a time long before, when my best friend Carol O'Malley and I had opened our own animal hospital. Carol lived down the block from me in Jersey City. Her folks, custodians of a four-story apartment building, were saving for the day they could buy a house of their own with cash. In the meantime, the two-bedroom apartment in the rear of the basement made do for Carol, her sister Diane and their parents.

To enter the basement, I had to walk down three steps from street level and press the bell at a heavy wooden door, which I did most school mornings and throughout the summers for years.

Inside the basement, along one wall, wooden slats partitioned off stalls used for tenants' storage. The first stall was empty and faced the street. On the moldy rug that covered the concrete floor, Carol and I had cared for a litter of abandoned kittens we fed with baby-doll bottles. A small crate, lined with towels, served as their bed.

In our ten-year-old minds, we were "animal doctors." We wrote "Animal Hospital" with bright blue crayon on a large piece of cardboard and shoved the sign through the bars on the window. The bottom of the window was eye-level on the inside and level with the sidewalk on the outside. We could survey only the feet of passersby.

One day, the neighborhood boys found four abandoned baby birds. They crouched down and pushed them under the bars through the open window.

"You got an animal hospital so take care of the birds," one boy ordered us though we screamed at them to stop.

The birds chirped and hopped on the dirty rug. The boys' raucous laughter filled the room as Carol and I scurried to gather the birds up before the kittens mauled them. I had a crush on one of the boys, but at that moment I hated him for putting the poor little birds at risk.

"Go to hell!" I yelled at him.

I felt a chill sweeping through my body. Not only had I cursed, I had condemned a child of God to go to hell. I had no way to take the words back. I just had to wait for God to strike me dead. When He didn't, I went home to dinner, and Carol had chores to do.

After a couple of days, we both had red blotches on our legs from the fleas that leapt up from the rug like popcorn kernels on a hot skillet.

We pulled the sign from the window.

We had relocated the birds to Carol's back yard, but what happened to the kittens? I wanted to believe Carol's mother had found what we were up to and stepped in to care for them.

Why did this memory resurface now? Did my clinic on the tenth floor resemble the basement "hospital," an inadequate environment with amateurish signage? Did Mattie and Mary remind me of Carol and me—well-meaning but inept? Taking care of Angelika seemed like delaying the inevitable. What would happen if she became ill over a weekend when the clinic was closed? Shouldn't she be in a nursing home? It wasn't my decision, since Ronnie and Antonio Sanchez kept abreast of Angelika's situation. I didn't need to get involved and I didn't want to get involved. However, I had a nagging sense I would get involved.

11

Visiting Ms. Henry

My last job had taken me four miles into the tranquil western suburbs. My commute, now eight miles, took me east. The panoramic view of the city skyline intensified as I drove through the assemblage of neighborhoods along Chicago Avenue.

At first, on nearly every block, storefront churches with hand-painted shingles mingled with ramshackle stores and boarded-up houses. In spite of the religious presence, crushed beer cans and liquor bottles littered the streets. After the church scene, neat brick bunga-lows emerged, with occasional Mom-and-Pop delis, their windows and doors covered by iron grates. Most mornings, I spotted a woman in a babushka sweeping the trash in front of her house into the street.

Soon storefronts outnumbered homes. Signs in English, Polish, and Spanish appeared. A full-size statue of a horse with a multicol-ored blanket across his back and a sombrero on his head stood in front of a clothing store. Later in the day, lively Latin music blasted from a loudspeaker mounted over the door.

The aroma of baking bread wafted into my car long before I came to the Polish bakery. As I turned into the narrow side street, I could see shadows of people clustering inside. Probably men in suit jackets and women in long, dark dresses—fresh from attending morning Mass at Saint Boniface Catholic Church—holding a number from the red dispenser by the front door and waiting their turn. I avoided the crowd, preferring to stop on my way home, hoping one babka would be left to bring to Mom.

One last turn after the bakery and the twenty-story high-rise emerged. After wedging the Datsun into a tight parking space across the street from the building, I always looked for the only two air conditioners in adjacent windows to pinpoint the Senior Clinic.

The elevator opened onto the tenth floor. I crossed the hall and unlocked the clinic door. The view of Chicago's skyscrapers through the smudged casement windows invariably overwhelmed me—so much so that I rarely noticed the battered desk, mismatched chairs, and worn linoleum floor anymore. The residents on our side of the building were treated to a view rivaling that of the pricey downtown condominiums on Lake Shore Drive!

I had scheduled myself to visit Ms. Henry to make sure that her medication was working. While I knew home visits were invaluable, and I didn't hesitate making them whenever I thought it was necessary, I still bristled when Sam, Mattie or Mrs. R decided that I should check on a resident. I ignored the discrepancy in my own logic.

I jogged up the seven flights to Ms. Henry's apartment, stopping every other flight to catch my breath, smooth down my tight skirt, and tell myself what a good workout I was getting.

I heard a child giggling as I stood outside Ms. Henry's door. Delilah let me in. Ms. Henry sat at the kitchen table with a toddler on her lap. His stubby fingers held half a hot dog.

As I passed Delilah, she said, "This is my son, Calvin."

Calvin slid off Ms. Henry's lap and ran on tiptoes to his mother, who settled him on her hip. He burrowed his head into her shoulder.

Ms. Henry patted the chair next to her. "Calvin's just shy. Come on and sit down."

"How's the foot?"

"Fine. Don't hurt no more."

I noticed a large bowl loaded with pill bottles at the edge of the table. I decided to inspect the foot first, then ask about them.

Ms. Henry kicked off her slippers. The right foot was cool to my touch.

"Looks great. Doesn't mean it won't flare up again. Sometimes other medicines can make uric acid build up in your blood. That's what causes gout. You did tell me you weren't taking any other medicine, right?"

Delilah reached over and shoved the bowl with the pill bottles toward me.

"This here is her medicine. She don't have no money to get them refilled, so she don't take them."

Ms. Henry gazed down at the table.

"Is this true, Ms. Henry?"

Calvin squirmed down his mother's body. His little feet hit the floor and he scooted toward the bedroom. Delilah followed.

"All I got is Social Security. It don't go far enough to pay rent, buy food, and get medicine, too," Ms. Henry said. She pulled the bowl closer, spilled the bottles onto the table.

"I was takin' some of these for sugar and high blood."

Delilah reappeared, cradling Calvin. She rocked from side to side while Calvin's eyelids fluttered closed.

"I worry about her not takin' her medicine."

Now seemed a good time to ask about Delilah's connection to Ms. Henry.

"How are you two related?"

"Delilah here is no kin of mine," Ms. Henry said. "She the house-keeper sent by the city."

Ms. Henry turned toward Delilah, and gave her a warm smile. "No kin of mine ever had such a good heart and care 'bout me the way Delilah do."

Was Delilah as dedicated as she appeared? It would help if she were involved in Ms. Henry's care.

"Well, I tell you what," I said. "Let's get you back down to the clinic. I can examine you, do some blood work, and start you on your medicine again. As you know, we have medicine in the clinic that you don't have to pay for. How does that sound?"

Delilah didn't give Ms. Henry a chance to speak.

"Sounds good. When?"

After we settled on a time, I left with a list of the medications that Ms. Henry had been taking.

Back in the office, I couldn't stop thinking about the two women. I knew that housekeepers funded by the city weren't allowed to bring children on the job. Yet Ms. Henry didn't mind. In fact, she seemed to enjoy having Calvin around. I wouldn't report it. I'd just keep my eyes open. Older folks were ripe for scams. You couldn't be too sure.

12

Dr. Braun Returns

Ingrid Braun dropped her purse and lab coat on a chair in the waiting room, and hung her silk jacket on the coat rack. She had just returned from a month-long trip.

"Before you inform me of what has been happening in the clinic, I need to do one thing."

She sauntered into the exam room. Her wool skirt and white blouse with a bow at the neck clung to her lithe figure. She slipped off her high heels and stepped on the scale.

"I didn't gain a pound," she said, showing her even white teeth—all capped, if I had to guess.

I had been so immersed among the bland elderly women in the building that Ingrid seemed to sparkle, resisting the inevitability of a dreary old age. She had to be in her seventies. Short salt-and-pepper hair feathered her face. Black mascara and liner highlighted her dark eyes, red lipstick tinted her lips, and pink blush powdered her cheeks. Of course, one thing Ingrid had, which the rest of the women who came to see me at the Senior Clinic didn't, was money.

As if on cue, Priscilla Hungerford appeared.

"So how was China?" Priscilla asked, sitting down next to Ingrid. Her tailored outfit complemented the doctor's. They could have been heading out to lunch at Marshall Field's Walnut Room.

Priscilla, a psychiatric social worker, had worked part-time at our high-rise before the Senior Clinic opened. A grant from Chicago Mental Health Services supported her visits to seniors who were a "danger to themselves or others." She also had a private practice in the Magnificent Mile, a classy area in downtown Chicago. She didn't report to me, but stopped in the clinic when she wanted me to examine someone she was following. And now she was here to see her friend, Ingrid Braun.

"Tell us," Mattie said as she shuffled in through the open clinic door.

Mary, trailing behind her, pulled the door closed. The women settled down to hear Ingrid's account of her trip. Mrs. R leaned across her desk, grinning.

The bright April sun warmed the reception area. I chose a chair next to Mrs. R's desk. As the ladies chitchatted, I scrutinized the group. They all had to be twenty years older than I, except for Priscilla, who had at least five years on me. At forty-two, I was the baby. Not only did I take care of old folks, they surrounded me in the office.

After Ingrid shared details of her vacation, she slipped on her lab coat, pulling her stethoscope from her purse. Pricilla, Mattie and Mary left the clinic while I trailed behind Ingrid to the exam room and closed the door, taking the chair beside the desk.

Ingrid secured her purse in the bottom drawer of the desk and took a seat. With her hands folded on her lap, she gazed at me over half-frame glasses. An aura of camaraderie connected us. We had first met when I interviewed for the job, and right from the beginning I felt we would work well together. She would see patients in the clinic on Monday afternoons only. But she was available to me by phone whenever I needed to contact her. As my collaborating physician, she and I shared responsibility for the same caseload of patients.

"We're getting new patients every week," I reported. "Some days are more quiet than others, but that gives me a chance to work on organizing the clinic."

I didn't tell her I was running up and down the stairwells pursuing emergences that never materialized. Then I mentioned Angelika.

"There's a lady who lives on the fourth floor that Mattie and Mary visit. The other residents of the building call her the Pigeon Lady. Her real name is Angelika Moustakas."

I had already decided to tell Ingrid about Angelika since someone might drop her name at one of our team meetings. I wanted her to know that she needn't get involved in Angelika's care since Sanchez seemed to have taken her up as a special project. I had been trying not to get involved, at least until the previous week, when Mattie told me Angelika had tripped and hurt her ankle.

When I arrived at Angelika's apartment to assess the injury, I couldn't help but notice how thin she was getting. Her usual laconic manner had deepened further to a nod here, a grunt there. Her ankle was swollen, warm, and painful. Money from Angelika's funds paid for a taxi. Mary accompanied her to the hospital for an x-ray.

Angelika had difficulty walking even though the x-rays were negative for a fracture. Who was going to follow up on her limited mobility? I didn't think Mattie or Mary would notice subtle fluctuations in Angelika's health status, and Ronnie and Sanchez came only at random times. I had taken the walker we kept in the clinic for her to use and called the Visiting Nurses' Association to arrange for nursing aides to come for eight hours on both Saturday and Sunday when no one from the clinic was around. If Angelika started to spiral down-ward, how long would her money hold out?

Ingrid suggested that I do a complete examination on Angelika, something I had been avoiding. "Do as much of a work-up as she will allow you to do."

I restrained my displeasure in Ingrid's directive. *Damn.* But in no way would I challenge her so early in our relationship.

Out in the reception area, three of Ingrid's regular patients were having a lively conversation. They had arrived early. During their appointments with Ingrid, she would tell them that they would see me for their care from now on. She would see them if and when I felt that their health problems had became so complicated that a doctor needed to weigh in.

Ingrid called after me.

"Marianna, I forgot to give you some prescriptions."

I watched as she signed along the bottom of each script. She handed me almost half a pad. Since she didn't date any of them, they would probably last months.

I shoved them into my lab coat pocket.

"Thanks." I wouldn't need to bother Sanchez for signed scripts even though he no longer required me to document the drug, dose, and patient.

The next day when Mattie stopped by the clinic, I asked her when would be a good time to visit Angelika.

"I'm going to do a physical and enroll her in the clinic," I said.

It was the last thing I wanted to do. But I had a nursing student shadowing me that day. And the clinic was slow. Sue would learn from observing a physical exam, regardless of how inept I appeared, since it would be the first physical I had done in a patient's apartment.

"Anytime you want. She's already had her breakfast. The door's unlocked," Mattie said.

Sue stepped into the elevator first, carrying a bedpan and a paper bag with the vaginal exam equipment. I had my nursing bag over my shoulder.

"Why a bedpan?" Sue asked as the elevator doors closed.

"If you are doing a vaginal exam on a bed, the inverted bedpan keeps the woman's pelvis from sinking into the mattress and making the cervix hard to see," I said. "I hope it works since I never used the bedpan trick before. I recently read about it in a nursing journal."

Angelika sat in her usual spot at the kitchen table, her injured ankle wrapped in an ace bandage, the walker by her side. She nodded agreement to the exam. How much did she understand? Was I taking advantage of this sick old woman just to demonstrate a physical exam to Sue and gain experience for myself? The ethical question didn't stop me from forging ahead.

I figured I could do most of the exam while Angelika sat.

First, I set up my equipment. Since I had a student with me, I had an obligation to demonstrate "clean technique" learned in my Public Health Nursing program.

Taking a couple of sheets of newspaper out of my bag, I spread them over the table, and placed my bag on top. The nursing bag had been born a diaper bag. The stethoscope and blood pressure cuff fitted into a compartment probably reserved for extra clothing, and the disposable gloves were bundled into a side pocket. Paper towels and a bottle of liquid soap slipped neatly into the diaper section. The removable pouch for baby lotion and burping cloths was perfect for blood tubes, needles, tourniquets, and alcohol sponges. I viewed the reincarnation of the diaper bag as a symbol of my ability to cope in the not-for-profit and under-funded clinic.

I took out the soap and paper towels along with the equipment I planned to use: stethoscope, reflex hammer, and thermometer, and placed everything on the newspaper—a "clean field."

When I was ready to leave, I would wipe off the equipment before putting it back into the bag. I would wash my hands one last time, and toss the newspapers and solid paper towels in the trash.

I unbuttoned Angelika's housedress. Sue watched as I pressed the stethoscope's diaphragm under Angelika's thin cotton slip, and checked her reflexes with the rubber hammer. The rest of the exam, including the Pap test, would have to be done lying down.

In the early eighties, Pap tests for women and rectal exams to check prostate glands for men were a standard part of the complete physical. And all patients newly enrolled in the Senior Clinic received a complete physical. Most of my patients told me that it was the most thorough exam that they had had. The "laying on of hands" during a new-patient visit seemed to develop a bond between us, and promoted trust. I wasn't sure what I expected would happen after I examined Angelika. I didn't expect to find anything significant. But I would be honoring Ingrid's directive.

"Angelika, let's get you over to the bed, it's easier to examine you there."

B. J. started to jump about in his cage on the dresser as Angelika shuffled into the bedroom with the walker, limping on her swollen ankle.

"What a cutie!" Sue said. B. J. twittered loudly.

Before Angelika sat on the bed, I took off her housedress. When I lifted her slip I found that she was wearing a diaper—not unusual for older women to protect their clothes from leaky bladders. The diaper was stained with dark yellow urine—she needed to drink more fluids—and streaks of blood. I locked eyes with Sue and shook my head indicating I had no intention of discussing this in front of Angelika.

I tossed the soiled diaper on the floor and snatched a towel to protect the clean bedsheets before she sat down.

Angelika lay in the bed with her hips elevated on the upside-down bedpan. Sue shone the flashlight over my right shoulder. The sweet musty smell of blood mixed with a rotting odor made me think Angelika was decaying from the inside out. I hoped to get this procedure over with before both Sue and I succumbed to the stench.

A blockage prevented me from inserting the speculum into her vagina. Maybe she had a tumor or had had a hysterectomy.

"Hand me the cotton swab," I asked Sue. When I removed the swab, it was covered with blood.

Sue and I cleaned Angelika up, put on a clean diaper, and left her resting in bed. Mary would come by soon to give her lunch.

Out in the hall, Sue coughed repeatedly. Her previously rosy complexion has taken on a light green hue.

"Not too pleasant, was it?" I asked.

Sue juggled the paraphernalia she carried to free one hand in order to search her pocket for a tissue.

"How sad." She coughed a few more times. "What's wrong with her?"

"Not sure, except now I know she's bleeding vaginally."

Before Sue could ask what I was planning, I added, "I'm just going to watch her. She already told us she didn't want anything done."

But I had no intention of watching Angelika. I planned to contact Sanchez and Ronnie about this latest finding. She was their responsibility, after all.

13

Resurrecting Old Problems

One Friday when I returned home from work, Annie stood in front of the open refrigerator, a container of milk in her hand. Her straight black hair flipped like a wave as she turned her head to greet me.

"Hello, Mom Crane."

"We still have some of that chocolate cake left over. It'll go well with the milk," I said.

Annie's plaid skirt dusted the floor as she bent down to search. The stove, cold and silent, indicated Mom had remembered not to cook dinner.

Jeannine surfaced from the basement, the sound of the TV drifting up behind her.

"Can Annie have supper with us?"

"She won't want to stay when she hears what we're having."

Dead silence.

"Geppetto's pizza."

Their giggling exploded about me.

Doug was over at his friend's house again. Avoiding his grand-mother, no doubt.

Mom was in her room, avoiding Annie. I knocked on her door hard enough to compete with the boom of the TV. I knocked again. When she turned down the volume, I yelled at the closed door.

"Are you going to join us for Geppetto's pizza tonight?" Then warning her, I added, "Annie's staying for dinner, too."

"No!"

Normally, I would have cajoled her. *Aw, come on, Mom, you love Gepetto's pizza. We're going to get stuffed spinach and a thin-crust pepperoni.*

Before I left for work that morning, Mom had complained again about the children's friends eating our food.

"You're not the protector of the pantry," I told her, surprising myself at the anger in my voice. "Jeannine's and Doug's friends are welcome in our house. I'll worry about the food."

Her expression turned stone hard.

I should have remembered she would still be angry. I stared at the closed door for a minute before walking away.

Mom didn't come down for pizza and sequestered herself in her room over the weekend, refusing to join us for meals. The children expressed concern.

"Nana wants to be in her room alone. She'll come out when she's ready to come out," I said. "Don't worry about her starving; she has opportunities to raid the refrigerator when we're all gone from the house."

Sunday night, I confided to my husband, "I'm not participating any longer in my mother's and my historical game. When I say something she doesn't want to hear, she's offended and angry, slipping into silence. After I apologize, we're fine until the next time she becomes displeased. Well, no more, Ernie. From now on, if she wants to be miserable, let her."

Monday morning, Mom sat at the dining room table reading the *Chicago Tribune*, pink chenille robe covering her pajamas. Her large-boned hand brought a slice of toast, loaded with orange marmalade, up to her mouth while her eyes scanned the comics. I surmised that she had ended her self-inflicted confinement because she believed it was time for me to say I was sorry.

"'Morning," I said as I made my way to the coffee pot. She grunted and continued reading. I slid a part of the paper to my side of the table before I sat down.

"Do you have something in mind for tonight's dinner?"

She hesitated a few moments before lifting her head.

"I was going to make spaghetti with meatballs."

"Good."

I sipped my coffee while I read the news. I knew the rules to this game only too well: the first one bringing up the disagreement lost. I clenched my jaw in determination, unsure of what had stiffened my spine. But this time I wasn't losing.

I drove to work feeling proud of myself for not falling into my old habit of apologizing. While Mom and I didn't continue our disagreement, we hadn't resolved anything. So I didn't lose, but I didn't win, either. I had just postponed the inevitable.

14

Confronting Sanchez

M attie and Mary routinely checked on Angelika before they went
home at the end of the day, but that Friday, I volunteered to look
in on her.

The moment I opened Angelika's unlocked door, the heat of the
apartment, mixed with the same rancid odor, sent me into a coughing
jag. Damn the CHA management for not putting thermostats in each
unit. It was entirely too warm.

Angelika sat slouched at the kitchen table. I called her name but
she didn't move. Instead, B. J. chirped a greeting from his cage in the
bedroom. Standing over Angelika, I saw globs of undigested food on
the front of her housedress and clinging to the hairs on her chin.

"Angelika, how are you? What happened?"

She didn't move. I shook her shoulder. She grimaced. Had she had
a stroke? I carefully scanned her face.

"How are you?" I repeated.

Still no response.

Her mouth was not drooping to one side, nor were her arms limp when I moved them. My fingers searched her wrist for a pulse. It was rapid but regular. Maybe it was the heat?

Damn. Damn. Damn. When did she get like this? Obviously, her condition had slipped downhill rapidly. What should I do? Return to the clinic and call 911? Whatever had happened should be evaluated in the emergency room. She needed to be admitted to the hospital where she would be tucked between clean, white sheets with around-the-clock nurses.

I stood by Angelika as my heart rate and breathing returned to normal. I couldn't ignore the fact that Sanchez, Ronnie, Mattie, and Mary had been looking after Angelika before I started at the clinic. They invested time in her care and they didn't want her to go to a hospital. And Angelika didn't want to leave her apartment. She wasn't my patient, yet I had no choice but to clean her up even though it was after five and I would be late picking up Jeannine from the orthodontist.

I opened the window a crack, slipped off my suit jacket and rolled up the sleeves of my broadcloth shirt. Filling a plastic basin with warm water, I parked it on the table.

"Angelika, I'm going to clean your face."

She seemed not to hear me but you never could tell.

The washcloth loosened the crusted plaques from Angelika's chin and they floated onto her lap.

"How about we get this dirty dress off of you?"

I slid my arms under her armpits. I braced myself to hoist her up so I could shimmy the dress over her hips. I tugged. She sat. Without her cooperation, I couldn't budge her. Putting Angelika in bed would make it easier to change her.

"Angelika, you're going for a ride."

I tipped her chair toward me, gripping the back with one hand and holding on to Angelika's boney shoulder with the other so she wouldn't fall off, and scraped the chair along the vinyl floor. Sweat dripped off my forehead, and my damp shirt stuck to me. I shoved the chair parallel to the bed. B. J.'s cage clattered as he jumped from perch to perch, cheering me on.

I pulled down the top sheet. A stench surged from the mattress. I stepped back to catch my breath. I stripped off the bottom sheet to find the mattress stained with variegations of color from bodily fluids, mainly blood. I quickly remade the bed using a plastic garbage bag as a barrier between the mattress and the clean sheets as Angelika sat slumped in the chair.

Bracing myself to move her onto the bed, memories popped into my head of transferring fellow student nurses in and out of hospital beds in the nursing lab while stiff-lipped instructors judged our technique. I pulled my straight skirt up over my thighs so I could widen my stance. With my knees bent and my arms under hers, I heaved Angelika up off the chair. Although we pivoted smoothly, she landed on the bed with a thump. My nursing instructor would have made me do the transfer over.

Angelika whimpered as I struggled to undress her. Shoulders, ribs and hipbones stood out prominently. Bright red blood stained her diaper.

After I changed the diaper and put on a clean nightgown, Angelika appeared comfortable. A pillow wedged under her back would keep her turned on her side. In this position, she wouldn't aspirate if she vomited again. Before I left the bedroom, I slid my wrinkled skirt down over my hips, dumped more birdseed out for B. J., and refilled his water.

In the kitchen, I pressed my ballpoint pen carefully over a paper towel as I wrote a note to the nursing aide who was scheduled to come the following morning. I was happy I had hired the aides before Angelika started on this downward spiral.

Angelika has been vomiting. Feed her soft foods. No liquids. There is pudding in the fridge. Feed her slowly when she is sitting up. Watch she doesn't choke. Don't bother to feed her if she is not hungry. I left a couple of quarters for the aide to use to wash the sheets in the building's laundry room.

Rolling down the sleeves of my soggy shirt, I shut the window, grabbed my jacket, and closed the apartment door behind me.

Angelika's body odor filled the interior of the car. I rolled down the window to let the wind blow away the stench. For some reason, I couldn't drive home. I made an illegal U-turn on busy Ashland Avenue and headed to the Family Health Center.

I pulled up in front of the one-story brick building. Before I got out of the car, I scrutinized the streets for boys ducking behind parked cars or running out of the alley.

Back in November, I had left the main center in the late afternoon after interviewing for the Senior Clinic job and had walked past clapboard houses with shabby sofas, tricycles, baby carriages, and toys crammed onto the porches, all evidence of the recent influx of young Mexican families into the neighborhood.

Back in the car, I put my purse on the floor, and locked the door before I drove down the narrow one-way street. I hadn't noticed the group of teenage boys congregating on the corner until they jumped into the roadway just a few feet from my car, hurling rocks at a second gang who popped out from behind parked cars farther down. A surge of adrenalin tightened my muscles, sharpened my vision, and caused my heart to beat so fast I could hardly catch my breath. I gripped the steering wheel and veered sharply to the left into a narrow alley.

Just as I exhaled after avoiding the gang fight, more boys ran toward me. I gunned the engine and flew past them as they plastered themselves against the alley walls. They defiantly scowled at me. I prayed not to get a flat speeding over the garbage-strewn cobblestones with my wheels jouncing up and down. At the end of the alley, I slowed to a stop before inching my car into rush-hour traffic.

The crowds of shoppers, bright streetlights, and other cars jostling for space on the road formed an aura of safety around me as I headed home. Soon the prickly sensation on my skin began to fade.

At the dinner table, I discussed my interview but kept my encounter with the gang to myself.

✳✳✳

Now I tramped into the quiet building, hoping Sanchez would be working late. Most of the staff had left. I followed the noise of the spinning centrifuge to the lab.

Driving over, I had whipped myself into a high level of agitation over Angelika's condition. "Is Sanchez still here?" I asked the tech. She pointed down the hall. I found him sitting at a desk in one of the exam rooms, a stack of patient charts in front of him. His lab coat hung over the back of the chair with a stethoscope dangling from a pocket.

"Hi," I said to alert him of my presence, and launched into my speech.

"I just came from Angelika's apartment. She may have had a stroke, and she's bleeding more. She vomited sometime today." My voice was loud and raspy. No patients were around, and I didn't care if any of the remaining staff heard me.

"What kind of half-baked care is she getting? It's just a matter of time before she aspirates and dies."

Sanchez turned in his chair. A frown pleated his dark, handsome face.

"What do you want to do?"

I screamed in my head. *What do I want to do? Are you kidding? She's not my patient. You're the one who comes over and checks on her. You support Mattie and Mary hovering over her, spending time with her.*

I shouted down at him, "She can't just rot in that apartment. She needs to be in a hospital."

He placed his pen down on the desk.

"That's not what she wants, is it?" he said calmly. "When I first saw Angelika, I wanted to put her into the hospital, too, to figure out what was going on. Angelika said 'No.'" He paused, watching my reaction.

"She knew she wasn't going to get better. She wanted to stay in her own apartment."

I didn't want to hear his words. His courteous demeanor sounded condescending and only made me more irate. I breathed in deeply, trying to control myself.

"Of course the hospital's not what she wants. But what she has now isn't adequate," I said.

I flopped down in the chair by his desk and blinked back the tears. By God, I wasn't going to cry in front of this man. He waited while I composed myself.

"I just can't stand to see her like this," I said, finally.

"If she did have a stroke, there's nothing we can do but keep her comfortable." He leaned closer to me. "I think we both want the same thing for Angelika."

Do we? I didn't want to admit he could be right.

✷✷✷

With my purse in the trunk, the doors locked, and the windows rolled up, I drove home along Chicago Avenue on a stretch of road notorious for "smash and grab." My mind replayed the conversation with

Sanchez. We had argued back and forth, neither giving in. Finally, I realized it was useless to demand that Angelika be admitted to the hospital. Hospitals didn't necessarily help folks die comfortably.

I tried to be alert to my surroundings as I passed clusters of young men congregating on street corners and lazing on steps in front of rundown houses, but my thoughts drifted back to Angelika. Slowly, I began to realize that by not wanting to get involved in her care, I had compromised her welfare. Sanchez was right to ask me what I wanted to do. I was the coordinator of the clinic. Mattie and Mary reported to me. I had abdicated my responsibility by letting them take charge, even if they were doing what Angelika wanted. How could they do a good job without some direction? After all, neither woman had a medical background.

What troubled me most, though, was that a doctor had to remind me of what I knew nurses did best—speaking up for a patient when she couldn't speak for herself. I had always prided myself on supporting my patients in the past. But right from the start, I hadn't thought of Angelika as my patient. Maybe because everyone fussed over her, I decided to ignore her. It wouldn't be the first time I had exhibited contrarian tendencies.

Starting Monday I would take responsibility for Angelika. If she was to remain in her own apartment, I would have to do something about that mattress.

15

At the Deli

As I crossed over Austin Boulevard, the divide between Chicago and Oak Park, the air seemed to lose its dusty haze. I took the first parking spot I could find on a side street near the orthodontist's office and raced around the corner. I spotted Jeannine's bright blue jacket. Her dark brown ponytail whipped back and forth as she searched for my car among the others zipping along the main drag. Annie leaned against the window of Erik's Deli. My remorse at being late eased a bit in seeing that Jeannine had a friend with her.

Annie's dark almond eyes spotted me first.

"See, your Mom's okay."

"Sorry to be so late," I said slightly breathless from dashing up the block.

"What took you so long, Mom?" Jeannine said as she ran up to me, hugging me tight. Her hair tickled my nose.

"Work." As usual, I didn't choose to explain. To divert any questions, I added, "Let's get something sweet."

There was nothing like Erik's made-on-the-premises pastry to waylay worry.

The girls ran ahead to find a table in the crowded deli while I fell in line to place our order. Rather than a slice of warm apple strudel and decaf, what I really needed was a long, hot shower to wash away Angelika's stench on my skin and clothes, followed by a glass—or two—of Merlot.

The line advanced slowly. My mind was back at the clinic. How would I find Angelika on Monday morning? While I thought about possible scenarios, a stately woman with short bluish hair, pearl earrings, and a long herringbone coat interrupted my thoughts. She had been motionless before the pastry counter for a long time. Her head started to bob ever so slightly. Her body swayed with greater and greater velocity—until she finally toppled backwards into the arms of a policeman who stood behind her. They both slid to the floor in slow motion. The other customers silently circled the duo, giving them space as if being on the floor was a common occurrence.

My mind juggled the pros and cons of intervening. He was a policeman. Surely he could handle the situation. I had had enough of sick old ladies for one day. My daughter didn't need to worry again where her mother had gone while I tackled another crisis. After a few seconds of watching the young policeman do nothing but stare at the woman, I pulled out of the line. *Damn.* I knelt next to the blue uniform. "I'm a nurse."

"I was just watching her. I knew she was going to fall," he said, excited to find himself in the middle of a medical emergency.

Then the old lady's face, heavily dusted with powder and rouge, started to twitch and contort. Her tongue twisted. Her eyelids fluttered. Saliva dripped from the side of her mouth.

"I think she's having a stroke," I whispered to the policeman. "Call 911."

He eased the woman's head onto my lap before he rose from the floor. I unbuttoned her coat and watched her chest rise and fall irregularly. A musty, old-lady smell arose from her. My fingers slid on her cool, clammy skin until they found a strong but uneven pulse on the side of her neck. I wouldn't need to start cardiopulmonary resuscitation—yet. I slipped off her glasses and placed them in the brown leather bag that had fallen on the floor beside her. Her tongue started to gyrate and shoved out a pair of slimy dentures, first the top, and then the bottom. I managed to grab a tissue from my coat pocket just in time to catch them as they tumbled from her mouth. The customers continued to circle around us at a respectable distance, observing quietly.

A siren wailed in the distance, becoming louder and louder until it halted in front of the deli. Through the large windows, I saw a white truck, *Oak Park Rescue Squad* printed on the side. The policeman directed two men in dark blue shirts and matching pants toward the deli. Wheeling a stretcher between them, they made their way through the crowd.

One of the men hoisted a small green oxygen cylinder from the stretcher and placed it on the floor next to the woman. Before he knelt down, I eased her head off my lap. He checked for a pulse at the side of her neck. While he turned on the flow of oxygen, slipping a clear plastic mask over her mouth and nose, the other man flattened the stretcher to the floor.

"Are you going to start an intravenous drip?" I asked. "Or strap her to an electrocardiogram?"

Both ignored me.

From the stitching on their pockets, I noted that the men were from the fire department. They had no other equipment with them other than the oxygen tank. I sat back on my heels and kept silent as they lifted the woman onto the stretcher. One of the fellows tucked a faded yellow blanket around her, and buckled her in. They raised the stretcher and rolled it toward the door.

I snatched the woman's purse from the floor; shoved the dentures inside and struggled to my feet, hampered by my tight skirt. I rushed to catch up with the stretcher. They didn't slow down as I flung the purse onto the woman's thighs. I watched as they loaded her into the back of the truck. What had just happened? It was inconceivable to me that they had done absolutely nothing to stabilize her.

Nothing.

Back inside the deli, I was still shaking my head when a woman with the deli logo on her apron touched my arm.

"Thank you so much for helping that poor woman," she said.

Then the policeman edged up to me.

"Thanks for calling 911," I said. "But they didn't start an IV. Didn't do an EKG."

"They aren't trained as paramedics, they're firemen from the rescue squad," he said. "But with all the taxes we pay, you'd think this town could afford a real ambulance service."

The siren wailed away into the evening air.

Jeannine rushed over to me, breathless.

"Mom, I wondered what happened to you. I thought you were the one hurt on the ground! Then I got close enough to see what was going on."

Poor baby, another scare over her mother. I hugged her close.

Huddled in a far corner of the deli, the girls planned their weekend while my coffee cooled. I wondered about the woman who had left on the stretcher. With no immediate medical intervention, would she be alive by the time the rescue squad reached the hospital?

Then I wondered again about Angelika. How long would she live?

16

New Clothes, Old Mattress

With my backpack slung over one shoulder, I maneuvered Jeannine's single mattress down the side stairs, careful not to get tangled up in my new swirly cotton skirt. Over the weekend Jeannine and I had visited the Futon Factory in Old Town, finally buying a futon covered with an orange flower motif that she had been asking for. Afterward, she helped me shop for new clothes: loose blouses, full skirts and flat shoes. My Evan-Picone suits would hang in the back of my closet until I could decide where to donate them.

The Monday morning sun hid behind dark clouds. Better not rain on the mattress. I had nothing to protect it. With the mattress squeezed onto the back seat of the car, I drove to work.

The rain began as I entered the building. With the mattress against the elevator wall, I rode up to Angelika's floor. The nursing agency hadn't phoned me over the weekend, so I figured Angelika must still be alive.

I didn't bother to knock. Holding the door open with my foot, I dragged the mattress into the apartment.

Mattie stood by the table folding a bed sheet.

"What's this?" she said, staring at the mattress.

"How's Angelika?"

I wanted to know how Angelika was before I answered Mattie. I turned into the bedroom. Angelika sat in a chair beside the bed while Mary combed her stringy hair.

"How are you feeling, Angelika?" I said.

Her head slowly nodded and maybe, just maybe, I saw the corners of her mouth move. Okay, she had a smidge more spark than she had last Friday, but there was no denying she was slowly wasting away.

"Angelika seems so weak this morning," Mattie said, entering the bedroom carrying a stack of clean linens.

"We had the toughest time getting her up and washed," Mary said as she stroked Angelika's arm.

"You didn't want to get out of bed this morning. Isn't that right, Angelika?" Mary exuded maternal warmth even though she had never borne children of her own. Mattie, on the other hand, had nine kids.

"She's not eating," Mattie said with a shake of her head, as if Angelika had made a deliberate choice.

"When I came down here last Friday, she didn't look so good. I thought maybe she'd had a stroke," I said.

Mattie inhaled deeply and held her breath for a few seconds before exhaling noisily. Mary's hand went to her heart. I had forgotten they have been sharing morning breakfast with Angelika for months. I made a mental note to share my assessments of Angelika more frequently in order to prepare them for her ultimate death.

"I was glad I had already scheduled the nursing aides to come over the weekend." I turned to Angelika. "Since you don't want to go to the hospital, we'll just keep a close eye on you here. Okay?"

I couldn't tell whether she nodded.

"It's a good idea not to force her to eat if she doesn't want to. Careful with liquids. Give them to her slowly and watch that she doesn't choke," I said to Mattie and Mary.

Both women listened silently. Even B. J. stopped hopping about and angled his head in my direction.

"And by the way, when I was here on Friday I noticed her mattress was stained with blood."

I dropped my backpack on the floor next to Jeannine's mattress.

"Over the weekend my daughter got a futon, so she doesn't need this anymore. It's in good condition."

After we exchanged mattresses and made the bed, Mattie said, "I'll ask Luther to take this old mattress away. Let's just leave it out in the hall."

As I left the apartment, I overheard Mattie. "She brings a mattress on her back! Did ya notice her outfit? She's gonna fit right in after all."

While I didn't know I was still on probation, it was nice to hear.

Later that day, as I sat in my office waiting for my first patient of the afternoon, the phone rang. It rang several more times before I realized Mrs. R was probably in the bathroom.

"VA hospital. Marianna Crane," I answered. Oops, not anymore. I quickly corrected myself. "Senior Clinic."

"Hello, my friend."

His familiar voice made my throat tighten. *How in God's name did he track me down at work?*

"Mr. Foley. How are you?"

"Not good. My wife died. She died a month ago." He began to sob.

Eddie Foley, a frail man with thinning white hair and a perpetual smile, had been one of my favorite patients at the VA. He often spoke of his wife and adult son.

"They mean all the world to me. I don't need no fancy vacations or new cars," he had said. "I'm happy as long as I got my family."

I reached for a tissue from the box on my desk, and mopped the tears dripping down my cheeks.

"Mr. Foley, I am so sorry."

Mr. Foley had been a butcher for over fifty years. One day he suddenly developed swelling and redness of both hands.

"Acute arthritis," Leon Logan, my doctor-boss had said. "While this is common with butchers who handle cold meat, it's unusual for it to occur for the first time so late in life. Let's put him in the hospital so the Rheumatology staff can learn from him."

I worried that Mr. Foley might catch a nosocomial infection, a new term in the eighties for hospital-acquired illnesses where many patients became sick from microorganisms contaminating stethoscopes, food trays, and health worker's hands.

Many died.

When I couldn't convince Dr. Logan not to admit him, I tried to dissuade Mr. Foley.

"You don't have to go into the hospital. The Rheumatology doctors want to see what has happened to you but there are textbooks they can read, you know."

"I'll do anything to help Dr. Logan and the other docs. If they can learn from me, I'll go into the hospital."

Damn.

The battery of tests and invasive procedures the doctors put Mr. Foley though had caused dehydration and weight loss. I walked into his room trying not to show my anger as I studied his labored breathing. He had developed pneumonia. A plastic bag hung from a pole dripping saline and antibiotics into his skinny arm. I sat down on the side of his bed and leaned close to his ear.

"Mr. Foley, you had better get well, your wife and son want you to come home." He smiled weakly. "You can do it."

Maybe I was cheering him on so I wouldn't live the rest of my life with his death on my conscience. I had let Dr. Logan get his way with little resistance. I should have tried harder, and vowed I would never be such a pushover again.

Three days later Mr. Foley was sitting up in bed reading a newspaper. The IV was gone.

"The docs say I'm a walking miracle. I go home tomorrow."

And he did, with another week of oral antibiotics. Home to his family.

While Mr. Foley continued to sob, Mrs. R shuffled through the door.

"Your patient is here," she said and laid the chart on my desk.

"Mr. Foley, I'm so sorry, I can't talk. I have a patient waiting."

"Oh, Doctor Crane, I shouldn't have bothered you," he replied, voice cracking.

I could never get him to stop calling me *doctor*. "You *are* my doctor," he would say. "And my friend."

"Mr. Foley, give me your address. I'll come and visit you."

I sensed him breaking into a smile. I wrote the address down and slipped the paper into my skirt pocket.

At that moment, I missed my old patients, the familiar routine, the well-equipped exam rooms, and the adequate supplies.

Before calling my patient into the exam room, I slipped into the bathroom, and splashed cold water on my face, blotting it dry with a coarse paper towel.

17

Planning the Funeral

Each Monday at noontime, before Ingrid Braun's afternoon clinic, we locked the door, sat in the waiting room and conducted our team meeting. Priscilla had started attending. That particular Monday, she showed up with a cloth lunch sack and thermos. Ingrid sipped a cup of black coffee. Mrs. R sat at her desk crunching on her lettuce salad. Mattie and Mary sat closest to the door so they could grab their purses after the meeting and, as usual, rush to a neighborhood restaurant for lunch.

I led the meetings. We discussed general business before talking about the most troublesome patients. That day I reported Angelika's decline, mostly for Ingrid's edification. She sat in her lab coat with her thin, shapely legs crossed, intent on what I was saying.

"She's getting weaker and the bleeding continues," I said.

I put my hot dog down on the wad of paper towels covering my lap. Before the meeting, I had driven to Donald Duk's on Ashland Avenue for french fries and a Chicago hot dog with everything on it, my once-a-month grease fix. I wiped my mouth with a flimsy paper napkin.

"I just increased the nursing aides to come on weekday evenings. We still don't have night coverage, but at this rate, I'm worried we'll spend all of Angelika's money in no time."

"I know that Delilah, Gladys Henry's housekeeper, would like to make extra money," Mattie said. "Maybe you could ask her to help with Angelika."

"Sure, good idea, I'll go up to Ms. Henry's after the meeting and see if Delilah's there."

I was pleased how easily we were working out details of Angelika's care.

"What'll we do when Angelika dies? I mean, will she have a funeral?" Mary said.

I popped the last bite of hot dog into my mouth. *A funeral? Since when does a clinic arrange for a funeral?*

Ingrid responded before I could finish chewing.

"I suppose we have the responsibility to see that her remains are appropriately disposed."

Maybe Ingrid had a point. I waited to see where this conversation was going.

"I have an idea," Priscilla said.

She screwed on the top of her thermos and slipped it into the lunch sack, placed the sack on Mrs. R's desk, and rearranged her pleated skirt before she continued.

"Let's use Dabrowski."

"Who's Dabrowski?" I asked, wiping the grease off my hands with a paper towel.

"He owns the funeral home just around the block," Mattie said. "Dabrowski does all the Polish funerals in this building and most of the others."

"Some of the residents pay him in installments. Some have been paid up for years," Mary added and then put a chubby finger up to her cheek. "You know, I have a dress in my closet that doesn't fit anymore. I'm gonna bring it in for Angelika to wear."

Mattie's forceful personality usually overshadowed Mary's. But slowly, over time, Mary had shared parts of her life that exposed a resilient core. A few years ago, her husband had had a heart attack in bed, and died in her arms. As if that wasn't enough trauma, soon after that Mary came home from work to discover an intruder raping her invalid mother, whom he had shoved onto a radiator. She died of burns a week later.

When Mary came to FHC to volunteer, Karen recognized her value as a Polish translator and put her on the payroll. The neighborhood had a large concentration of Poles, many of them speaking only Polish.

But Mary's strength, as far as I could see, was her graceful ability to play second fiddle to Mattie while still keeping focused on her job. I never saw her irritated or upset by Mattie's strong persona. Mary was diplomatic and seemed comfortable with herself, not needing to compete with Mattie.

I rinsed off my hands in the kitchen sink as the women chattered about funerals, wakes, flowers, and all the trimmings, details I hadn't thought of. But then I had never before arranged a funeral. And I couldn't think of any reason to object.

Back in my seat, I said, "I'll contact Dabrowski."

But first I visited Ms. Henry.

Delilah opened the door. Evidence of lunch in progress lay on the kitchen table: bowls, coffee cups, slices of bread, a half-full glass of milk. A large pot on the stove gave off a sweet earthy scent—maybe vegetable soup? Healthier than the greasy hot dog and fries I had just wolfed down. Through the wide-open bedroom door, I saw Calvin curled up asleep on the double bed.

"I won't disturb your lunch. I just have a proposition for Delilah."

Delilah cried when I told her Angelika had no family or friends to care for her—just the staff from the clinic, and the nursing aides I had hired.

"I just don't know how she can be without kin," she said as she wiped her palms across her eyes.

Delilah agreed to watch Angelika during the night.

"Calvin can sleep here with Ms. Henry. Then I can check on Angelika fine," she said. "Sometimes Calvin and I stay over anyway."

On top of bringing a child to work, if Delilah's boss found out she also stayed overnight, she would surely lose her job. I prayed no busybody in the building would report her. With Delilah working nights, Angelika would have almost twenty-four-hour coverage.

Although I offered Delilah less money than I paid the agency, she said, "That's a lot more than I make working for the city."

She would start that night.

18

The Video Guy

The next day, Karen Cranston called me from the main center.

"Meet me at the Pigeon Lady's apartment in twenty minutes."

Angelika's door was ajar, and I heard Mattie talking. A deep voice interjected *wow* and *oh, my*. I pushed the door open. Karen was standing in the kitchen beside a tall man with a large camera case slung over his shoulder. Mary was sitting down at the table. Mattie leaned against the kitchen sink. Angelika dozed quietly in her bed.

Mattie noticed me first.

"Marianna, I was just tellin' Chris here about how we found Angelika."

She was in her element: telling stories.

"This is Marianna Crane, the coordinator of the Senior Clinic." Karen said, and turned to the man. "This is Christopher Colford. Chris works in the media department at the University. He came here to see what we are doing at the clinic. He wants to do a video on Angelika."

Chris was good-looking in an all-American-preppy way, much younger than any of us.

"Karen told me about the clinic," he said, even white teeth sparkling. "I'm impressed. Not the usual set-up. Angelika's would make a great human-interest story."

I wasn't surprised to hear Karen promoting the clinic. She was the director, after all. She had developed FHC into an independent, full-service entity, opening two satellite clinics as well, one for seniors and one for teens. Just recently she'd succeeded in getting a government grant to support and expand services. Besides being married and pregnant, Karen was going for her Ph.D. in nursing.

Chris scanned the apartment.

"What a great set-up this is. The video will be awesome."

Chris was all youthful enthusiasm and naiveté. Didn't he feel some reluctance to film a dying woman who, if she had been alert, would probably refuse the intrusion? However, Karen probably supported the video to give FHC some publicity. Who was I to second-guess her strategy?

"I'm going to take Chris up to the clinic and then show him around the building," Karen said. Turning to Chris, she added, "I'll give you the clinic number, Chris, and you can call Marianna to arrange for a time and day to start videotaping."

Somehow Angelika's dying had taken a voyeuristic turn I hadn't imagined. I felt uncomfortable in being part of that, but I wasn't sure what to do about it.

19

Dabrowski's Funeral Home

The traffic light on wires across Chicago Avenue rocked in the April breeze. I walked toward the sign above a storefront in the middle of the block: *Dabrowski's Funeral Home.* I pushed open the heavy wooden door. A tinny bell announced my arrival. As my eyes adjusted to the dimly lit hall, I barely made out an older woman in a wheelchair propelling herself soundlessly toward me.

"Good morning," she said. "Can I help you?"

A blue dress covered her ample body. White elastic stockings compressed her thick legs. Her rouged cheeks, pink lips, and empathic expression anticipated my bereavement.

"I'm Marianna Crane. I run the Senior Clinic in the CHA building around the corner on North Noble. I'd like to talk to Mr. Dabrowski about funeral arrangements for one of my patients."

After I said these words, I wanted to laugh. Here I was planning a funeral for a patient from a clinic where people were supposed to get well.

But the woman didn't seem to catch the irony.

"I'm Stanley's mother. He isn't in the office right now."

I must have looked disappointed, because she added, "Follow me, I'll get him on the phone."

She rolled over the thick carpet past a couple of darkened rooms. The third room had an open casket with a bald man decked out in a pinstriped suit. Hating wakes, I turned away. The muted silence, sickening floral scent, and vacant folding chairs facing the coffin made me edgy and breathless.

I had attended three wakes in my life. Jimmy Costello had had a brain tumor and died when he was six. He lived with his parents and three older brothers down the block from me in Jersey City. In the summer at dusk, skinny elbows resting on his knees, Jimmy sat on my stoop with the other kids as I faced them and told spooky stories before the streetlights went on and our mothers called us home.

Carol and I walked down busy Montgomery Street by ourselves to the downtown funeral home. We were eleven. One glimpse at Jimmy's little body in a dark blue suit lying so still in the ornate coffin made me bolt outside to sob in the cold night air. I had never expected children could die, especially such a sweet kid like Jimmy.

The old lady who lived two houses down from me died just after Jimmy. All of us kids called her The Witch. Whenever she swept her sidewalk, we raced back and forth past her house until she chased us with her broom. We delighted in hearing her yell, "Get off my property, you ragamuffins!"

After she died, Carol and I attended her wake, entering her dark frame house for the first time. We tiptoed up the creaky steps to the second floor where The Witch lay in an open casket. Carol gripped my arm when she spotted The Witch sitting in one of the folding chairs— a replica of the figure lying in the coffin. We had never known The Witch had an identical twin.

My grandfather died when I was a freshman in high school. He was a gentle man who spoke soft words with a thick Italian accent. When I was little, he would pull me onto his lap and call me *bambino*. His mustache tickled my face. He always smelled of pipe tobacco and garlic. My cousins and I gathered around him with outstretched hands after Sunday dinner when he handed out nickels and dimes. No one I loved was supposed to die.

From then on, I avoided wakes.

***

Mrs. Dabrowski turned into the last room, picked up the receiver on a huge mahogany desk, dialed, and handed it to me. After I introduced myself, and stated my mission, I added, "We would like something modest. Our patient doesn't have much money."

Stanley Dabrowski's baritone boomed in my ear.

"We could pick her up—Saint Elizabeth Hospital could pronounce her—we'll embalm her, lay her out, do a run to the cemetery for 475 but you got to buy the burial plot."

What do I know about buying burial plots?

"The Greeks are tight, but the Catholics would give you a break." He paused. "Take this number down."

Mrs. Dabrowski, who could hear her son's voice, handed me paper and pen. I leaned on the desk.

"Ready."

"Call the public administrator's office after she dies. They will come out to her apartment and search for money, bank accounts. If they find any, it will go to the burial expenses. If not, Cook County Morgue for thirty days, if no one claims her then to Potter's Field."

"But we have money to bury her," I reminded him.

"Right," he said, and continued to tell me the public administrator would also search for any relatives that Angelika might have.

I worried that a cousin could come forward after Angelika's death and question my using her money for the in-home care or for arranging her burial. In the short time I had worked at the Senior Clinic, I had met some strange, greedy family members.

Good God. What have I gotten myself into here?

We agreed to meet the following Monday to finalize the arrangements for the funeral. "If she dies in the meantime, call me first, then the public administrator."

Back outside in the bright sunlight, I retraced my steps back to the clinic. I never thought that my responsibility for Angelika would extend beyond her death. But rather than feel anger at finding myself planning a funeral, I was enjoying the novelty of the task.

20

To the Bank

It was only three blocks to the bank. If I could cash Angelika's two Social Security and three Supplemental Security Income checks, I would have over $700 in my purse. With that much money on me, I preferred not to walk.

Before we had left for the bank, I wrote on the back of the checks "payable to Marianna Crane" and then signed Angelika's name. I can't say "forged" her name since I didn't have a copy of her signature in the first place.

"I sure hope you get the cash," Mattie said, tucking her polyester skirt under her legs before she closed the car door. "How can we pay for the nursing aides and the funeral if we don't get this money? They better not give you no trouble."

I clutched the wheel. How surreal all this seemed. Cashing some dying woman's checks so she could stay in her own apartment, and then when she did finally die, she could have a wake—and a funeral. Since Angelika had money, there was no reason she had to go to Cook County Morgue and then to Potter's Field, Chicago's cemetery for the indigent. Of course, someone had to make the arrangements, and the payments—and it so happened that was me.

"Mattie, I'm going to hand over the checks to the bank teller, and wait to see if *she* has any questions rather than explain anything first. The less we say, the better." I had planned that if the teller questioned me, I would ask to see the manager. He could call Karen at FHC to vouch for me.

Inside the bank, three people waited in line for the one cashier behind tall iron grates. I predicted the young female teller with short dark hair and a pleasant countenance wouldn't think twice about cashing the checks and handing over the money. Even so, my stomach gurgled noisily.

The line moved too slowly. I needed some distraction to quell my nerves.

"What are you doing for Easter?" I asked Mattie a bit too loudly.

A youngish man turned from the cashier, slipping an envelope into the back pocket of his jeans. Now only two were in front of us.

She detailed an elaborate feast. After all she had had nine children.

"Our Easter is going to be quiet. Just my husband, kids, and my mother."

After the second person in line turned to leave the bank, the last guy squeezed a fat beige sack under the grate. The teller opened the bag and pulled out a thick stash of bills. She counted. *Good lord, how long will this take?*

Finally, we were at the window. "Good morning," I said as nonchalantly as I could, and slipped the loose checks to the teller.

"I want to cash these, please."

I hoped I didn't sound nervous. The teller gathered up the checks. She inspected each, one by one, separating them with the brown rubber cap on her index finger. I waited for her to look up at me, ask my name, ask me to show identification, then say, big-eyed, "Please wait while I call the police." Instead, she punched in the amount of each check on an adding machine, ripped off the tally, and set it front of her. My stomach gurgled so loudly I was sure she heard it.

"Do you want any hundred-dollar bills?"

The teller didn't look up. Had she already decided that the two of us, one middle-aged white and one older black woman, were totally harmless and ordinary?

It took a second for the question to register.

"Sure. Give me four hundreds and the rest in fifties and twenties."

Ouch, did that make sense?

The teller used her rubber-tipped finger to count out each bill. I turned to Mattie to distract myself.

"What are you having for dessert?" I said.

While I tried to appear interested in Mattie's description of her Easter menu, I kept glancing at the teller. She shoved the bills into an envelope, folded over the flap, and guided the envelope under the grate toward me. I willed my hand not to snatch the envelope too quickly.

I dared not count the money in the bank, and I dared not peek at Mattie. I just hoped her face was as expressionless as I was trying to make mine. I put the envelope into my purse, then pressed it tightly to my side. If anyone snatched my purse, I'd come with it.

Once we were in the car, Mattie laughed in relief.

I wasn't ready to relax. I looked out the back window as we drove away, expecting to see the bank manager running into the street, waving his fist at us and shouting "Stop! Thieves!"

21

Good Friday

The stiff, new bills from the bank were stuffed inside a locked metal box that was shoved behind the disposable gloves on a shelf in the kitchen cabinet. Because the box was out of sight, I believed the money was safe. The truth was that anyone could open the kitchen cabinet, move the gloves aside, grab the box, and run out of the clinic. Nevertheless, for now I had money to pay for Angelika's care, and even for the funeral.

Angelika had sunk into a coma. It wouldn't be long before she died. She was in no position to be a star in her own documentary, and I was relieved when Karen called to tell me Chris couldn't do the story.

"Our lawyer said it's questionable that Angelika is able to give informed consent," she said.

Questionable? I thought, but didn't reply. Instead, I asked Karen for the lawyer's name and number. How convenient FHC had a lawyer. I planned to contact him to ensure I was on legal footing in arranging for Angelika's funeral.

I had canceled the nursing aides. Delilah planned to spend the Easter holiday with Ms. Henry so she could just walk down the staircase and visit Angelika at intervals throughout the day and night. "Just keep her comfortable," I told Delilah.

Before I left for the three-day weekend, I stopped at Angelika's to give Delilah last-minute instructions. Delilah met me at the door, flushed and grinning.

"What's going on, Delilah?"

"Who is that gorgeous man?" she asked, leaning her mouth close to my ear and jerking her head towards Sanchez. He was sitting on the side of Angelika's bed dressed in chinos and a polo shirt, his stethoscope planted on her chest.

"Dr. Sanchez," I said.

"He's a doctor?" she tittered.

Was this the same Delilah who cradled her toddler and rocked him to sleep? Who managed Ms. Henry's medications? Who assured me she was very capable of caring for Angelika? This unprofessional behavior made her a ditzy preteen. I put my arm around her shoulders, steered her out to the hall, and closed the door behind us.

"Delilah. Have you ever seen a person die?"

Her chortling stopped and her mouth dropped open.

"Angelika's dying and may very well die this weekend," I said with such an air of confidence, I impressed myself.

I had seen people dead in hospitals. Mostly after failed CPR. Once, I found an older man sprawled on the floor, dead of an apparent heart attack. He was ice-cold and stiff. No one was around to call a code. I had never orchestrated a home death, but there I was, the expert.

Delilah hung on my words.

"To be sure she's dead, listen for her breathing. Sometimes, when people are dying, their breathing is irregular, and there are long intervals between breaths. You can put your hand on her chest, and leave it there for a while to make sure her chest isn't moving."

Delilah slumped against the wall as if facing a firing squad.

"Are you going to be all right with this, Delilah?" I asked. Her head bobbed forward.

"We want Angelika to be comfortable. Keep her clean. Turn her in bed every two to three hours."

Delilah stared at me, waiting for my next words. This was what I wanted: her full attention.

"If she dies, call me. Then call Mr. Dabrowski at the funeral home. He'll send an ambulance for her body. Stick around until he picks her up. I'll write down the phone numbers and put them on the kitchen table. I'm sure Molly Flanagan will let you use her phone."

Molly, a wiry, eighty-year-old woman with an Irish brogue, lived next door to Ms. Henry. She often dropped into the clinic to socialize rather than to seek care. She didn't take medication, and rarely complained of aches or pains. I was sure she would let Delilah use her phone for clinic business.

Delilah and I plodded back into the apartment. Even though the brown spots from the bird droppings still dotted the walls, there was now a medicinal smell to the place. The stove, refrigerator, and kitchen cabinets gleamed a bright white. A sturdy trashcan with a pedal to open the top had replaced the cheap plastic wastebasket. Clean white linen and towels were stacked on one of the kitchen chairs. The only sound cutting the stillness was the jingle of the birdcage as B. J. hopped about.

Antonio Sanchez wandered from the bedroom, slipping the stethoscope into his back pocket. Behind him, Angelika lay, as white as the sheets covering her. Her chest cycled up and down slowly. He shook his head. Up to that moment, I hadn't appreciated his genuine concern for Angelika.

He looked so sad that I walked up to him and put my hand on his arm and said, "We've arranged for Angelika's burial, so she won't go to Potter's Field. She has enough money for a wake, too." *Although I'm not sure who will show up.*

On Good Friday morning I was enjoying a second cup of coffee at my dining room table when Delilah called. Between sobs, she said she had just stepped into the apartment, and noticed Angelika was not breathing. She rushed up to Molly's apartment to call me.

"Delilah, you need to go back to Angelika's, and make sure she's dead. Remember what I said about putting your hand on her chest, and feeling for any breathing, any movement. What would happen if Dabrowski picked her up and she was still alive? Call me back."

"Yes," she whispered.

"Oh, and don't forget to take B. J. back with you to Ms. Henry's."

"Yes, ma'am."

I imagined Delilah creeping down the stairs to Angelika's, each step pounding more fear into her. Stopping at the door, terrified at what would be inside. Angelika sitting up at the side of the bed beckoning to her?

I could see Delilah slowly turning the knob and then the stuffy, stale odor hitting her nostrils. Delilah would force herself to focus on Angelika's bed once more. Would she feel relief if Angelika hadn't moved? Maybe she'd break into a sweat trying to gather enough gumption to place one of her little hands on Angelika's cold chest.

I felt sorry for Delilah having to touch a dead person. She certainly hadn't earned much money being on duty with Angelika for such a short time. I would slip her an extra twenty when I paid her on Monday.

Thirty minutes later, Delilah called back.

"Nothing. I feel nothing."

She was still sobbing.

"She's dead." More sobs.

I was surprised to feel tears drip down my own cheek.

"Delilah, you did a wonderful job. Thank you. Please call Mr. Dabrowski now. He'll tell you what time he'll come to pick up the body."

After I hung up, I called Mattie. The moment she heard my voice, she said, "Angelika's dead."

While my coffee reheated in the microwave, the phone rang. Dabrowski's deep voice asked, who would sign the death certificate?

"Dr. Sanchez," I told him. Dabrowski agreed to wait until Monday to call him.

And on Monday, I would tell Dabrowski we didn't have a cemetery plot.

22

Easter Sunday

Mom didn't even bother to ask me to go with her as she donned her coat and slammed the door to walk the two blocks to Saint Catherine and Saint Lucy Catholic Church. I sat on the sofa facing the large windows with the *New York Times* scattered next to me. To my left, Ernie lowered the magazine section and shifted in his favorite chair, an Eames chair we had bought for a pittance at a furniture outlet in the city several years before. We locked eyes briefly and went back to our Sunday-morning ritual.

I hadn't stepped into a church in years. The changes from the Second Vatican Council, a period of time between 1962 and 1965 when the Church's traditions were modernized, had had a profound effect on me. Practices that I was taught, beliefs I had to adhere to under pain of mortal sin, were no longer dogma. After being told to accept, unquestioningly, the mysteries of the Church, I felt I had been lied to both by the Dominican nuns who had taught me catechism in Saint Aedan's Grammar School and the Jesuit priests who gave the homily on Sundays.

I would be a hypocrite if I raised my children in the Catholic faith. No amount of Mom's ranting that her grandchildren should be enrolled in religious lessons could make me put my children into the arms of the same Church that had manipulated my conscience in my younger years.

Religion wasn't a big issue for Ernie. As he grew up, his mother dragged him and his two sisters from one faith to another as a serial social investment: Baptist, Methodist, and Episcopalian. In making moral choices, Ernie followed his conscience thereafter, while I struggled with the inevitable damnation of my soul to hell after each misstep in life.

"Guilt," he told me, "is a wasted emotion."

"Guilt," I replied, "is the glue of Catholicism."

When I had entered nursing school in September 1959, I carried with me a fear that I didn't possess the compassion needed to be a good nurse. Maybe that's why I went to Mass in the hospital chapel each morning, praying none of the Grey Nuns would notice that I didn't have the integrity to become a professional nurse, tap me on the shoulder, and tell me to leave.

When the nuns counseled that we, nursing students, were chosen by God to care for our less fortunate brothers and sisters, I replayed the episode that trigged a deep regret—I had abandoned a woman I was instructed to feed on my first day as a hospital volunteer when I was thirteen. That summer before Carol and I started high school, we sat on the edge of our chairs while a matronly woman behind the desk in the hospital's Volunteer Office surveyed us over the top of her glasses.

"It makes sense to start slowly. One day a week to help feed the patients lunch, then build up to three times a week."

We assured her we were more than ready to start at three days.

On our first day, and without any orientation, Carol and I were sent to different floors. A tall woman in a crisp, white dress, with an organdy cupcake cap perched on her head and a pleasant smile, walked over to me as I stepped off the elevator.

"So you are our new volunteer? I have just the patient for you to feed today."

I followed her stiffly as she led me down the hall and into a chilly room with white tile walls. A thin woman lay belly down on a stretcher.

"The floor is over-crowded, so we had to put her here in the Utility Room," the nurse said.

I later learned the Utility Room was where bedpans were flushed and dirty sheets tossed down the laundry chute. The nurse noticed me staring at the odd stretcher that seemed to have another stretcher suspended above it.

"We have her on a special bed," the nurse explained. "This top frame can be lowered down so we sort of sandwich her to turn her onto her back, and then to her abdomen again. We rotate her every two hours."

I had never seen such a contraption. It looked to me more like an instrument of torture.

The nurse put down the side rail, and slid the lunch tray closer to the woman.

"She doesn't speak English," she said, and abruptly left the room.

The metal chair clattered across the tile floor as I dragged it over to the stretcher. I sat down and shivered. I tried to tell myself that this was no different from babysitting.

"Okay," I said, trying to sound cheerful, "let's see what you have to eat."

The woman turned toward me, her dark eyes blank. A sour smell intermingled with the aroma from her lunch tray on the stainless-steel table.

I fed her slowly, alternating spoonfuls of soft mushy food and sips of milk from a straw, and watched for choking.

She ate hungrily.

"I hope you like vanilla pudding?" I didn't get a response. The nurse didn't tell me what language the lady spoke, not that it would've helped. I had only studied Latin.

Getting up from the chair, I wiped the lady's mouth with a paper towel. After I figured out how to secure the side rail, I paced around the room. Where was that nurse? The chilled air, the silent lady, the stench from the dirty linen and the bedpan hopper closed in on me.

I dashed into the hall. Avoiding the elevators and the nursing station, I ran down the stairs and out the emergency exit, not giving a thought to Carol, or what the lady at the volunteer office would think of me.

All the way home—and many times over the years—I pondered whether I was cut out to be a nurse.

★★★

All through my nursing career I had been incrementally shedding my Catholic beliefs. On this Easter Sunday, when again I didn't go to Mass with my mother, I believed my caring instincts were no longer dependent on a religious doctrine.

Yet, I couldn't deny I had shown little empathy for Angelika. In fact, I was relieved she had finally died, less because it had ended her suffering and more because I no longer had to organize her care.

However, the funeral still needed attention.

Mom returned from Mass, hung up her coat, and ascended the stairs to change into her housedress. I, for once, happily volunteered to assist her in the kitchen any way she would allow, just to be busy, and to avoid thinking about Angelika's funeral—and the lady on the strange-looking stretcher almost thirty years earlier.

23

Have Dress, No Plot

Stanley Dabrowski looked younger than I had imagined. A mop of sandy hair topped his baby face. I sat on one of three leather chairs in front of his desk, with Mary's red dress that Angelika would wear for the wake folded on my lap.

"We'll do a half a casket since we have no shoes or underwear," he said, reaching for the dress. "Leave that with me. My mother does the final preparations."

When I told him I hadn't gotten around to purchasing a plot, he said. "Cremation for 380 or embalm, visitation, and cremation for 500."

"By the way," I said as I signed the papers for the $500 package, "when I stopped by Angelika's apartment this morning, yellow police tape blocked her door. And a sign saying something about a 'Coroner's Case.'"

I had gone to check the apartment to make sure Delilah had taken B. J. back to Ms. Henry's place. I didn't expect to see Angelika's door taped shut as if it were a crime scene. I could only think that the ambulance workers who picked up Angelika's body routinely suspected foul play whenever a person died at home, and sealed off the death site. How would they have known that Angelika had died from natural causes? I had forgotten to call the Public Administrator's office as Dabrowski instructed.

Dabrowski raised an eyebrow and lunged for the phone.

"We need to get the Public Administrator involved."

Waiting for a connection seemed to calm him. He started joking with whoever picked up at the other end. When he hung up the phone, he said, "Someone from the Public Administrator's Office will come by tomorrow."

I remembered Dabrowski had said the Public Administrator would search for money, bank accounts—and relatives.

The next day the tape was gone, and the door to Angelika's apartment was ajar. A man with a crew cut and dressed in a dark suit knelt on the floor of the closet rummaging through Angelika's battered old suitcase. He was lucky Mattie and Mary had disposed of the dead pigeon.

The man on the floor kept shuffling items about. Another man ransacked the bedroom, pulling out the dresser drawers and dumping clothes onto the bed.

I didn't see B. J.

"Hello," I said. "I'm the nurse practitioner from the clinic. We took care of Angelika Moustakas."

Both men ignored me. Their indifference made me want to talk all the more, invade their space, make noise over their single-minded search. I jabbered on.

"We've arranged her funeral. Afterwards she'll be cremated."

The man in the closet sat back on his heels. He measured out his words in a low voice.

"Only a blood relative can sign for a cremation," he said flatly, not bothering to look at me.

He directed his attention back to the clutter strewn on the closet floor.

A weight fell on my chest. Oh my God. I ignored the formality of saying good-bye, and stomped up the steps to the clinic. Damn the lawyer and Dabrowski. My professional license was on the line. I wanted to shake these two men who were supposed to know more than I about legal issues. I only hoped I wasn't too late. Where was Angelika at this very moment? Maybe in the oven? Oh, wait. I remembered. We planned to have the wake first. My frenzy sputtered and slowed.

I rushed breathlessly past Mrs. R. In my office I picked up the phone, and called Dabrowski. He answered on the second ring.

"I can't sign for the cremation. I'm not a blood relative."

"I'll get back to you," he said, unfazed.

24

Retirement Party

"Thirty years with the CHA is enough," Sam Levy said with a laugh as we stood outside his office.

He patted his snow-topped head.

"I started out with dark brown hair. Time to go."

Earlier that day, someone had left a handwritten note on Mrs. R's desk inviting the clinic staff to Sam's retirement party. Contribution of five dollars per person requested.

I wanted Sam to hang around a little longer. Who would take his place? Maybe a by-the-book manager? Sam ignored some of the restrictive rules of the CHA and used common sense when enforcing others.

He had looked the other way as Mattie and Mary came and went into Angelika's apartment. Even if Angelika no longer angered her neighbors by tossing breadcrumbs onto the sidewalks around the building to feed the pigeons, they had still complained to Sam about the clinic staff helping her. How did they know that we were caring for Angelika? And who were *they*? Sam never shared names. The venom seeping from some of the old folks dismayed me. But Sam ignored their displeasure.

"Ya know," he had said, "if Angelika Moustakas wants to die in her own place, and you ladies can take care of her right up to the end, that's okay with me. You're doing a good job."

Even though at the time I was unsure if we should be investing so much time and attention on Angelika, I appreciated his support.

Two weeks later, at five o'clock, Mattie, Mary, Priscilla, and I locked the clinic door behind us, and stepped onto the elevator. The usually shabby room on the twentieth floor, with its only redeeming feature the large windows facing Chicago's skyline, had become a banquet hall. White cloths and flower centerpieces covered the tables. Women in fancy attire and men in suits and ties filled the room.

At first I didn't recognize the sixty or seventy guests as the stodgy, colorless residents of the building. Where were the dour faces I had seen in the hallways? Or in my own office as they complained of this ache or that pain? I had anticipated a brief good-bye party. The extravagant display astonished me. Plus the invitation hadn't mentioned formal dress. None of us had changed from our work clothes.

Charlotte Cook, a tall woman, elegant in a floor-length lavender dress, approached.

"Sam wants you all at the head table."

She led us to where Sam sat with a woman close to his age. To my relief, they both wore casual outfits.

Sam sprang to his feet.

"This is my wife, Beverly. Honey, this is the clinic staff I told you about."

Sam's wife exuded a sweetness that seemed a mismatch for the man I knew only as the overworked manager of a decaying building.

So Sam had a life outside of work. And he spoke about us when he was home. I wished I had gotten to know him better. Especially as I watched the residents coming to the table to wish him well. He hugged the women, none of them taking offense as he called them "Doll" and "Sweetie" and "Honey." They just smiled, fluttering their eyelashes. The men shook Sam's hand, and Sam patted their shoulders.

While we were still finishing dessert, someone clinked a water glass to hush the group. I recognized Hazel Gleason. One of few residents who had a car, Hazel charged her neighbors for transportation. Her pleasant manner and soft voice didn't suggest the scalper I had pictured. She spoke, as did several others following her, mentioning Sam's open-door policy, sense of humor, and fairness in solving problems. At a lull in the testimonials, Sam turned, jerking his head to the side as if he expected me to stand.

So I did. I remember saying, "Don't retire from life." I had just heard the expression on some inspirational TV show. Whatever else I said, I'm sure I was sincere. I liked Sam and was sorry to see him go. Priscilla and Mattie each said a few words, while Mary dusted crumbs from her lap and was passed over.

I was impressed that the residents had joined together to put on this shindig for Sam. I imagined the financially strapped CHA probably just had a luncheon at the main office, and gave him a certificate of commendation rather than a gold watch. I was embarrassed that I had planned to just drop in, and leave early. What a wonderful demonstration of appreciation for Sam's many years of service. His gesture of inclusion—asking me and the other clinic staff to sit at the head table—left me humbled. How could I have discounted the effect the Senior Clinic made in the lives of the elderly who lived in the building? And to Sam?

Someone had brought a radio. A Hawaiian melody filled the room.

One of the guests wandered into the middle of the floor and began to dance a hula. Others joined in. Sam grabbed my hand, and we wedged ourselves among the dancers. Jerry Johnson, mildly retarded, wiggled between us, gyrating and twisting with abandon. It was a raucous moment that transcended age and ability. Sam and I stumbled back to our chairs laughing as Beverly applauded our efforts.

Lilly Parks, a strikingly attractive woman in her seventies, stuffed her shawl down the front of her dress, and staggered about the dance floor on her matchstick legs as if she was going into labor. I had heard she kept a silver handgun in her sock, but that evening she must have left it at home since her slim ankles were surrounded only by her rolled-down stockings. She waddled around in the center of the room clutching her belly to hoots from an enthusiastic audience.

Skimming the sea of smiling faces, I wondered which ones had objected to the support the Senior Clinic had given Angelika.

25

The Funeral

D abrowski's voice boomed in my ear, "I'm waking her on Friday."
He had already told me he would handle everything—even the
burial plot. "Two to four in the afternoon."

Following the informal custom of the building, Mattie posted a
sign by the elevators noting the date, time, and place of Angelika
Moustakas's wake. As Priscilla said, how many people knew Angelika
was the Pigeon Lady? Who would show up?

Friday afternoon, Mattie, Mary, Priscilla, and I walked down the
hushed corridor of the funeral home. The thick flowery scent immediately set off my nerves. I didn't want to be there, but I had to see for
myself if we had gotten our money's worth. We passed several empty
rooms searching for Angelika—May must have been a slow month.
We found her in the last and smallest room.

The sight of two floral sprays on either side of the coffin stunned
me. Who had thought of sending flowers? Certainly not me.

Six women sat in the room. The two Greek sisters that had refused
to translate for her when Mattie and Mary thought Angelika spoke

only Greek sat primly on the aisle closest to us. Mattie pulled at my jacket until I bent toward her.

She whispered loudly in my ear, "Hypocrites."

I stared at the carpet, sure the women had heard. The third woman settled in front of the casket like a long-lost relative, her hands kneading rosary beads. She lived in the building but didn't come to our clinic. Who was the fourth woman in the chair by the wall? I gave Mattie a quizzical look. She shrugged her shoulders. The last two, Karen and Juanita, the nurse who had donated B. J., occupied the back row. They waved to us. Priscilla joined them.

Mattie, Mary and I stood in front of Angelika's coffin. She was exposed only from the waist up. Her skeletal hands crossed her chest and rested on the red dress Mary had donated.

Mary and I waited our turn as Mattie bent slowly to kneel beside the coffin. Silent and somber, she stayed there for less than a minute. When she was done, she pressed both hands on the padded rail and hoisted herself up with a muffled grunt.

Mary knelt next. She made the sign of the cross, and prayed silently before reaching into the coffin to finger the dress she had donated. What was she thinking? Had she worn that dress to a special celebration with her husband? The red dress may have elicited memories that would be buried along with Angelika. Mary made the sign of the cross again before she slowly raised herself up from the kneeler.

Then it was my turn. I knelt on the soft leather cushion, and inhaled the sweet powdery scent that oozed from the casket's satin lining. Since the coffin was on loan, I wondered how many other dead bodies had rested in it. Dabrowski's mother had dusted Angelika's waxen cheeks with pink blush, arranged her thin gray hair in a tight knot on top of her head, and disguised Angelika as a dowager. I missed the bandana.

Peering into Angelika's coffin I wondered if she had any awareness of the clinic's support, especially Mattie and Mary's attention. She might have spent her last days wasting away in her apartment with only her pigeons. I felt a sense of achievement that I'd orchestrated the wake and eventual burial, conveniently forgetting my initial reluctance to get involved.

Before I joined Karen and the others, I read the card attached to the spray of white carnations. "From the staff at the Family Health Center."

I had never thought to buy flowers. And if I had, would I have used Angelika's money?

The floral arrangement on the left had red and purple flowers I didn't recognize mixed with white carnations. The card was buried deep in the foliage. I wrenched it out trying not to snap off any blooms. A simple cross was embossed on the front. I opened it and read, "From Stanley and Sophie Dabrowski."

26

Pearlie Banks

One morning while I waited for the slow elevator, I noticed two women, one tall and lean and the other short and squat, at the far end of the lobby whispering to each other, and glancing my way.

I knew the tall one, Mabel Fitts, because she often stopped by the clinic to speak with Mattie, and occasionally to me. Her visits were brief and social. Mabel was in her sixties, her skin light mocha, and her figure curvy and sensual. The other woman looked at least ten years older, heavy-set with an indigo tint to her black skin.

Mabel shoved her friend toward me. I faced the elevator doors, bracing myself for whatever was coming.

"Excuse me," the woman said. "I'm Pearlie Banks." She extended a hand that felt like well-kneaded dough. In her other hand she clutched a baby food jar partially filled with brown liquid. Behind her I glimpsed Mabel ducking around the corner.

"I want you to be my doctor."

The woman sidled in so close to me that I had to step back to get a good look at her. She had an open, friendly face, and brown-stained teeth.

"I'm not a doctor, Ms. Banks. I'm a nurse practitioner."

"Don't matter. I want you to take care of me."

No one had ever walked up to me and asked me to take care of them. I felt flattered.

"I'd be happy to," I said. "If you already see another doctor, I'll need your old medical records."

Pearlie nodded.

"Stop by the clinic when you can. Mrs. R will help you get your records and make an appointment."

Pearlie strutted away.

Inside the elevator, I smiled all the way up to the tenth floor.

The next time Mabel Fitts dropped by the office, I asked why she didn't enroll in the clinic herself.

"I ain't got nothing wrong with me," Mabel answered. "No cause to be a bother to you."

"Ms. Fitts, it's my job to keep folks healthy. Besides, all women need to get some tests once a year, like pap smears and mammograms."

"I don't want no tests. If something's wrong, I don't want to know. No way."

She scurried out of the clinic without speaking to Mattie.

Pearlie showed up for her first appointment in a yellow print dress and orthopedic shoes. In one hand she carried a paper bag with all the medicines she was taking, and in the other, the baby food jar. When she sat down beside my desk, the skirt of her dress hiked up to reveal stockings rolled around garters below her knees. Judging by her thick ankles, the tight garters hindered the circulation to her legs.

From her records I knew Pearlie was seventy-two years old, overweight by fifty pounds, and had high blood pressure and congestive heart failure. Her doctor had prescribed digitalis and a water pill along with an antihypertensive. But in spite of the appropriate medications,

Pearlie made frequent visits to the emergency room when she had difficulty breathing.

"When I can't breathe too good, I takes a glass of 7-Up and I tosses in a handful of salt and drink it up."

I kept my face from showing any reaction to this appalling statement. The salt would attract water into her circulation. Her blood pressure would rise, and breathing would get worse, not better, but I wouldn't get any cooperation if I looked shocked or disapproving.

"When the 7-Up don't work, I go to the emergency room right away. Costs a bit of money. I asks Clara Gleason to drive me, and she gets five dollars. One time, I called the ambulance to take me."

She unscrewed the top of the jar, spit a stream of tobacco juice into it, screwed the top back on, and then wiped her mouth with a ratty-looking handkerchief she pulled out of her dress pocket.

"I don't like goin' to the hospital."

I wondered if her previous doctor knew about the salt and 7-Up. No wonder she had problems breathing.

"Let's see if we can keep you from having to go to the emergency room. Okay?"

"How we gonna do that?"

"Well, when you start to get short of breath, don't take the salt and 7-Up. You come right over to the clinic."

The way she leaned toward me, stock-still as if absorbing my every word, gave me the feeling she would follow my instructions—at least at first, and if I kept them simple.

"For the next few weeks, I want you to come every Friday afternoon so I can weigh you."

I picked Friday to catch any problem before the weekend when the clinic was closed.

Most of the folks who came to the Senior Clinic liked the attention, and didn't object to having their health monitored more frequently. We never billed over what Medicare paid so they didn't have to fork out cash for each appointment. If the patient was too young for Medicare we charged five dollars a visit. But we never charged for a weight or blood pressure check.

Before Pearlie left, I gave a short explanation of why salt didn't help her breathing, and cautioned her not to wear the tight garters. I would address her tobacco habit at another visit. I didn't want to overwhelm her with too many instructions at once.

Many of my patients did well from education, close follow-up, and noticeable improvements.

Would Pearlie?

27

Adopted Granddaughter

I took a large envelope from the wire basket on the kitchen counter and lifted out the packet of lab results. I had planned to review them for abnormalities. I was especially concerned that a new patient might have latent syphilis. Before I took this job, I would never have guessed how many of my elderly patients had a sexually transmitted disease.

I turned to the first page just as Mattie and Mary stomped into the room, planting themselves in front of me.

Without even a *good morning*, Mattie said, "Every time we go into Ms. Sims' apartment something else is missing." Anger clouded her face. "We just came from there. Now her good china is gone. That girl could be stealing from Ms. Sims to buy drugs."

"Ms. Sims calls her 'my adopted granddaughter,'" Mary said. "But we don't know how they know each other."

I laid the lab sheets on the counter.

Mattie and Mary had been bugging me ever since the floor captain, Charlotte Cook, pulled them aside to say that a young woman had begun visiting Ms. Sims, and soon after, things started to disappear from her apartment.

Bless those floor captains, most of them women, who kept watch over the people that lived on their floors. Some were better than others, but without them Mattie and Mary would miss lots of problems.

"I thought you told me Ms. Sims doesn't want you to do anything," I said. "She loves that girl, right?"

"Come on and just speak with Ms. Sims," Mattie pleaded.

Even after all we did for Angelika, who did not ask for our help, either, I still felt uneasy stepping in where I wasn't invited.

However, I had begun to realize that Mattie and Mary believed that my presence served as a "symbol of authority" and would add legitimacy to their involvement. I left with the women to visit Ms. Sims on the fourth floor—the Pigeon Lady's floor.

I would review the lab results later.

A petite woman opened the door and scanned me from head to toe. Mattie introduced me to Elsie Sims. She led us though the living room, past a sofa, an empty china cabinet, and into the kitchen. I made a mental note of the scant furniture.

Mattie, Mary, and I sat down at the polished wooden table. Paisley cushions were tied to the backs and seats of the chairs. In the center of the table a blue earthen pot held artificial daisies. We three sat while Ms. Sims stood, her knotted fingers gripping the back of the chair.

"What can I do for you ladies?"

She could have been royalty—her bearing aloof and distant—or she could have been wary of three intrusive women.

Mattie leaped in.

"Ms. Sims, tell Mrs. Crane about your granddaughter. What she's been doing."

Ms. Sims pulled her shoulders back.

"Why, that sweet girl is doing nothing but bringing a little sunshine into this old lady's dull days." Her eyes narrowed. "My word, what do you think my grandbaby is doing?"

Mattie shook her head in disbelief.

"Ms. Sims." Mattie's voice sounded more gruff that usual. "Your granddaughter is stealing from you. She's taken your things to sell. Just look around here."

Ms. Sims' body stiffened. "Nonsense," she said.

She stomped toward the door, and held it open for us.

"Well, that visit fell flat on its face," I said as we headed toward the elevator. "Ms. Sims is just not ready to give up on that granddaughter, is she?"

Mattie and Mary continued to hear from Charlotte Cook about the latest piece of furniture or knickknack that had gone missing. I pushed their updates into a faraway corner of my mind. Getting involved in these issues exhausted me, and I wasn't sure what I could do to make a difference.

A few weeks later, Mattie interrupted the quiet I enjoyed before the clinic officially opened for business. With a cup of coffee, I sat in the waiting room watching the sun glitter over the tops of Chicago's skyscrapers.

"I ran into Charlotte Cook a little while ago," she said, filling a cup from the coffee pot in the kitchen. She sat down across from me. I gripped my own mug tightly with both hands. "She told me Ms. Sims' granddaughter has a boyfriend."

"So? What's wrong with having a boyfriend?"

"Charlotte says they have a key to Ms. Sims' apartment. She watched them let themselves in."

"Ms. Sims probably gave her granddaughter a key."

"Charlotte says he looks like a hoodlum."

"Hoodlum? Huh! Well, it's what he does that counts. Not what he looks like."

Mattie ignored my argument.

"Then why did she give Charlotte money to hold onto?" She took a sip of coffee before she continued. "One hundred and eighty dollars."

She widened her eyes in emphasis, and said, "She told Charlotte to keep the money safe for her."

As I washed out my coffee cup, I gathered my thoughts.

Over the running water, I said, "Well, we can't do anything unless Ms. Sims asks us for help."

It was closing time when Priscilla Hungerford swept into the office, her long beige skirt whirling about her ankles. She stopped at the side of my desk, brusquely pushed up one sleeve of her white cardigan sweater, then the other, as if getting ready to fight.

"I just came from seeing Ms. Sims. It's a bad scene."

"What are you talking about?" I said. "How did you get involved with Ms. Sims?"

"Mattie asked me to see her."

Ah yes, I hadn't taken enough interest in Ms. Sims. Mattie and Mary generally avoided Priscilla, saying she was a bit too haughty for them, but now they had aligned with her. I was outnumbered.

"Ms. Sims' granddaughter and boyfriend were in the bedroom while I was there. The door was closed but you could guess what was going on."

Priscilla's stare could make me feel guilty even if I had no reason to be.

"The apartment is nearly empty." She paused, letting me take in the implication.

"I didn't talk at length to Ms. Sims with the granddaughter and her boyfriend there. I say YOU go back when they're gone. Maybe some-time tomorrow."

She said this with the authority of a commanding officer delegating orders to a flunky.

"I'll think about it," I said, not wanting to give her the satisfaction of my consent.

I watched as she swished out the door. Maybe she was right.

The next afternoon while I was with a patient, someone knocked on the examining room door.

"Mrs. Crane, can I speak to you for a minute?"

It was Mary's voice.

I excused myself, leaving my patient sitting on the exam table. Perspiration glittered on Mary's face as if she had rushed up the stairs.

"Mattie and me ran into Ms. Sims as she was coming back from the store. She says she's scared. We went back with her to her apartment. Her granddaughter and boyfriend weren't there. Mattie's still down with her. Can you come?"

I had already planned to visit Ms. Sims later in the day. It would be good to get this over with.

"I'll come down as soon as I finish seeing my patient." If Priscilla hadn't been off that day, I would've dragged her along.

When I knocked on Ms. Sims' door, Mattie opened it. Ms. Sims sat stiffly on one of two kitchen chairs left in the apartment. The table was gone. Her hands kneaded a flowered handkerchief in her lap and teardrops glinted off her dark cheeks.

Mattie—the protector and defender of those in need—walked to Ms. Sims and placed her hand on Ms. Sims' shoulder. Before I could say "Hello," Mattie spoke out.

"The granddaughter and her boyfriend are doing drugs. Robbing Ms. Sims blind. Selling her furniture. They go in her bedroom whenever they want. Do whatever they want."

Mattie's short, squat frame seemed to grow taller with her wrath.

As the air swelled with her words, there was nowhere for Ms. Sims, or me, to hide. Ms. Sims' shoulders shook as she muffled her sobs by pressing the handkerchief to her mouth. This time she didn't challenge Mattie's comments.

There was no way to deny something had to be done. I pulled the other chair close to Ms. Sims, and sat facing her.

"What do you want us to do, Ms. Sims?"

Mattie blurted out what Ms. Sims couldn't say: "Change the locks. Luther can do it. Just call him."

"Is that what you want to do, Ms. Sims?"

I heard a muted "yes" as she sobbed into her handkerchief again.

I pulled out my appointment book from the pocket of my lab coat, and opened it to the last page where I kept important phone numbers. I hoped Luther hadn't left for the day.

"Can I use your phone, Ms. Sims?"

While Luther set up his tools, Mary took my chair next to Ms. Sims and patted her arm.

Mattie left to visit Charlotte Cook. I stood by watching Luther as he quickly changed the locks. Clearly he had done this before.

Just as he was cleaning up, Charlotte Cook marched into the apartment with Mattie. Charlotte's slippers slapped the floor as she trod over to Ms. Sims, ignoring the rest of us. A stiff cotton housecoat covered her long, lean frame. She bent, and enclosed Ms. Sims with her skinny arms.

"There, there, Elsie, honey. Come on, pack a bag and stay with me tonight."

Charlotte turned to me. "This way she won't be tempted to let them trouble makers in when they come back."

Mattie, Mary, and Charlotte Cook all rallied around Elsie Sims. Even Priscilla saw the need to step in and protect her. In spite of my involvement in Angelika's care, I still hadn't acknowledged my respon-sibility to protect the safety of those so fragile, especially when they weren't asking for my help. Most times the patient didn't even know what they needed.

And I didn't know my mental block against taking action would come back to haunt me.

28

Thanksgiving

"Marianna!" my mother called from the kitchen.

I spread my open book face-down on the sofa. I shot an exasperated glance at Ernie as I rose. He put the *Times* crossword on his lap and scrutinized me. His facial expression seemed to say "Relax: don't let her get to you." Easy for him to be tolerant. She wasn't his mother. He wasn't a part of our long-standing dysfunctional relationship.

Mom insisted on a traditional Thanksgiving dinner even when Ernie and I didn't care and the children would just as soon have pasta with meatballs. While she assured me she could handle the preliminaries herself, I knew she would complain later of fatigue, insinuating that no one cared enough to help her—draping her martyr mantle over the whole family.

The oven door was open, emitting the luscious smell of roasting turkey. Mom handed me two oven mitts, and we wordlessly carried out the rote procedure. I pulled out the baking pan holding the ten-pound bird, then placed it on top of the stove, closing the oven door.

The drippings on the bottom of the pan spat and sputtered as Mom sucked them up with a glass bulb baster and squirted the liquid over the bird. Two more squirts, and she was done. She backed away as I replaced the turkey in the oven, returned to the living room, and waited for the next shout.

After dinner, I scraped the plates off, and Mom stacked the pots and pans in the sink. She liked to wash the dishes immediately after we ate. Before Mom came to live with us, the kids took turns setting the table and washing dishes. We didn't have an automatic dishwasher. Since Mom viewed the kitchen as her domain, she had taken over their chores as well. She wore her responsibilities like a badge of honor or a burden, depending on her mood.

Leaving the turkey carcass for me to dismantle, Mom sorted the leftover vegetables. After pressing the potatoes into a pie plate with a spatula, she took her anger out on the aluminum foil dispenser, ripping the sheet off with vengeance. As she worked, she criticized her grandchildren's friends.

"That Annie! She has her head in the refrigerator all the time. Eating our food. Doesn't she have any food in her own house? Tell her to go home and eat there."

I grabbed the turkey leg, and vigorously twisted it at the hip joint while blocking out my mother's words.

Then she stabbed at Ernie.

"That guy," she said, "has no respect for me."

I could see Ernie walking up the hall to the kitchen as Mom opened the refrigerator and placed the pie plate with the potatoes on the bottom shelf. The refrigerator door blocked Ernie from her sight as he stood at the entrance to the kitchen.

I froze in place while she continued to berate my husband.

"He could come and help in the kitchen once in a while, too. You should tell him to do that if he wants to eat. He needs to do his share of the clean up. He's a no-good, lazy loafer."

Ernie stopped, and stared at the wooden floor before he turned, and walked back down the hall.

Sadness enveloped me. Ernie had not only heard Mom complain about him, he had heard my silence. I didn't stand up for him. I didn't confront my mother.

Too quickly, I had forgotten my resolve to challenge Mom when she criticized my family. I had fallen into the old habit of my childhood when it had been so easy to ignore her while she griped.

At that moment, I vowed that I would begin to break that old habit, too.

29

Chicago Conference

"I'm so nervous," Mattie said to the standing-room-only audience.

Mattie stood on a stool so she could see over the lectern. Drops of sweat glistened on her dark forehead. The mike clipped to the collar of her blue dress amplified her trembling voice over the muffled sounds of traffic outside on Michigan Avenue.

"We found her sick in her apartment. She didn't have no relatives." Mattie was telling the story of the Pigeon Lady.

Mattie and I were speakers at a national convention held at the Congress Hotel for government-sponsored community clinics. In planning for the presentation, I had wanted the tale of the Pigeon Lady to show that our clinic did all kinds of non-traditional interventions. I asked Mattie to join me because her simple delivery and lack of professional posturing would best make that point.

Two weeks earlier, I wouldn't have bet that Mattie would agree to give this talk with me.

"You've talked in public before. You were a board member. In fact, you were the chair of the board."

"That don't count. That was way back when FHC first got started. Plus, I knew everybody on the board." Mattie frowned at me. "This is a big conference. I know none of these folks. And there are too many of 'em."

"You know the story of Angelika, and you're the best one to tell it. The audience will love you."

And they did. Men in dark suits, white shirts, and ties listened attentively. Women with coiffed hair and wearing pantsuits or dresses under suit jackets nodded their heads in empathy at the Pigeon Lady's plight.

Mattie shuffled the yellow pages of hand-written notes in front of her but didn't read them. Her cheeks rolled up into soft pillows crinkling her eyes. She spoke as if she was sharing a story with a neighbor at her kitchen table.

"We even held a wake," Mattie said, energized by the crowd's eager response.

A middle-aged woman in a plaid jacket seated in the front row dabbed the corner of her eye with a handkerchief.

When she finished, the audience clapped long and loud.

Mattie removed the mike, laying it on the lectern. She carefully backed off the stool, and climbed down the steps of the podium to join me in the front row. She beamed as she took her seat. I reached out and pressed her hand.

"Good job," I whispered.

My turn. I had given many talks before, so the packed audience didn't intimidate me. I started off by mentioning that the funeral director had returned the payment for the services, so we established the Angelika Moustakas Memorial Fund that supported the care we gave to the poorest of our patients. I omitted mentioning that the Public Administrator's Office found a bank account with a thousand dollars. Since no relatives had turned up, the money went into the fund, too. Who knew if someone in the audience might be related to Angelika? Or claim to be?

However, the rest of my nuts-and-bolts lecture paled in comparison to Mattie's animated talk. Dry, dry, dry, I thought as I heard myself drone on. Straying from the loose outline I had with me, an uneasy feeling crept over me. My words sounded conflicted. I was supposed to be saying the clinic was running efficiently and effectively. Instead I heard an undercurrent of criticism as I described how Mattie and Mary recruited patients for the clinic, and if they uncovered social issues they became mine to address, more often than not. I pushed myself to end on a positive note depicting all the health promotional activities our clinic supported—blood pressure screening, exercise classes, brown-bag lectures where the participants brought in all their medications so we could review what they took and give advice on effectiveness and safety.

Ending my talk, I asked, "Any questions?"

The woman in the plaid jacket, who minutes ago was moved to tears, raised her hand. I had a hunch I wouldn't like her question.

"How can you put so much time and effort into one patient—the Pigeon Lady? Aren't there so many more who need your services?" she asked.

An icy silence showered down on the room. Those leaning against the back wall appeared to straighten up. The folks smiling with delight as Mattie told about smothering the Pigeon Lady with care and concern, now seemed to glare at me. The spotlight made me dizzy. My face felt flushed. The woman had picked up on my internal conflict, which I hadn't realized I still had even though Angelika had been dead for eight months. I still hadn't condoned all the attention we gave her—just one patient. No rationale tripped off my tongue.

So I sputtered, and fumbled, and spit something out that sounded to my ears like a weak justification. Now I wanted to become invisible though the woman nodded as if I had successfully answered her.

Grateful she didn't continue to confront me, I took a couple of benign questions before walking off the podium to polite applause.

During the rest of the conference I was too busy replaying my dismal performance to listen to the other speakers.

Back at the clinic, while Mattie gloried in her successful presentation, I contemplated the dichotomy of my beliefs. Had ditching my high heels and Evan-Picone suits really altered me? Why hadn't my values changed with my choice of outfits? Why did I still resist following up on patients, like Elsie Sims, or even finding out what happened to Thelma Scruggs?

One thing I did know for sure: That day at the podium I was the emperor—without any clothes.

The following Monday while I was restocking supplies, Mrs. R told me that a Michael Foley wanted to speak to me. I froze in place as I suddenly remembered the piece of paper with Mr. Foley's address that sat in the top drawer of my desk. Ingrid was in the office seeing her last patient, so I took Mrs. R's phone, on which I had the forethought to put a long cord. Dragging the phone with me into the bathroom, I closed the door.

"Ms. Crane, this is Mike, Eddie Foley's son."

He sounded like his father.

"My father thought the world of you. So I wanted to let you know that he died last week. I guess he didn't want to live without my mother."

I slid down the wall onto the cold tile floor with the phone in my lap, shocked to realize that I never did visit Mr. Foley.

PART THREE
PLAYING SHERIFF

30

Intergenerational Love-In

Driving to work under the slate-colored sky past piles of sooty snow on the sidewalks took a toll on my mood. I hadn't seen the sun in days. February was my least favorite month in Chicago.

Inside the elevator I pressed the tenth-floor button, and had gone as far as the second floor when the doors creaked open. Mattie and Mary stood side-by-side, both wearing bib aprons over their dresses.

"Good morning," Mary said cheerfully.

Her sleeves were rolled up above her elbows. Her doughy white hand gripped a shopping bag stuffed with paper supplies.

"Today the daycare children are coming," Mattie said, her gruff voice jovial.

She shoved a shaky cart onto the elevator loaded with pots, pans, and a large coffee pot.

"What? Do you remember that we have the community health screening scheduled this morning?" I asked.

"Oh dear," Mattie said, her smile gone. "Guess we just forgot."

Mary mumbled, "Sorry."

I shook my head in disbelief. The two women were hosting a luncheon for the residents and inviting the children from a nearby daycare center. After lunch, the children planned to put on a little show. I supported their plan. Recent studies had shown that intermingling young children with the elderly benefitted both groups.

But Mattie and Mary had never told me the day. And this was the wrong day to be cooking for a luncheon when I expected them to help with registration.

We rode up in silence to the tenth floor. Before I stepped off the elevator, I turned. Did their gloomy expressions reflect shame for letting me down? I hoped so.

"We need to improve communication," I said, looking at each woman in turn before I walked into the clinic.

Laverne Weaver wheeled the old blood pressure machine out of the exam room. She wore a blue lab coat over a sweater and gray slacks. Silver clips pulled her thick hair back from her light brown face.

"I just met Mattie and Mary in the elevator. Today is the luncheon for the seniors and daycare kids."

I wanted her to join me in my exasperation. After all, I had hired her. She was a fellow nurse who, like me, believed patient care came first. Laverne made the routine home visits, did weight and blood pressure checks in the clinic, and conducted the community services I no longer had time for.

Instead of concurring with me, though, Laverne said, "We'll be okay. I'm sure I can get a couple of the floor captains to help out with registration."

We had put up signs in the neighborhood shops, grocery stores, and a notice in the Sunday church bulletin announcing free blood pressure monitoring, weight check, and glucose testing to be held that morning in the community room on the first floor. Since I had never organized a community health screening before, I had no idea how many would come. Thankfully, the Community Nursing Agency agreed to send two nurses to participate. The event would be good public relations for them as well as for as the Senior Center.

While Laverne collected her supplies for the screening, Rosie Fernandez watered the fern on her desk. The plant, and Rosie's appearance—long, dark hair, curvy figure, and a Hispanic flair for colorful dress—softened the institutional climate of the office. Rosie had replaced Mrs. R, whom I didn't miss. With Rosie and Laverne around, the clinic appeared more professional.

After shaking off my disappointment in Mattie and Mary, I remembered that Stella Bukowski was coming to the clinic. I had a non-paying faculty appointment at the College of Nursing. I gave occasional lectures and served as preceptor for nursing students. That day I was supervising a nurse practitioner student, Rita Wisniewski. Stella had agreed to let Rita examine her.

Stella used a three-prong cane to steady herself as she limped on her prosthetic leg into the exam room. She wore lipstick, and for a change her wig sat straight on her head. I was pleased but not surprised to see the effort she had made to impress. Although she always needed urging to come to the clinic when she was sick, and had refused to have health maintenance check-ups, she was more than willing to help educate a student nurse.

"Stella," I had asked her, "I have a nurse practitioner student who needs experience examining a patient. Are you interested in helping me? You are such a good example of how an older person can live independently."

Her ego sufficiently stroked, she agreed immediately. It didn't occur to her that I had found a way to give her a complete examination, including the routine tests she had previously refused.

I settled into a chair in the corner of the exam room, ready to observe Rita and Stella's interaction. My mind drifted back to the day I had first met Stella. I had been alone in the clinic when she rolled her wheelchair off the elevator and stopped in front of the open door. She peered inside, saw me, turned around, and careened down the hallway. *Where the hell was she going?* I took off after her. She braked at the end of the corridor. Trapped in a dead end, she sat in her chair, silent.

I bent down so I could see her face. "I'm Marianna Crane, the nurse practitioner. What can I do for you?" I said.

Stella concentrated on her hands gripped in her lap.

"Is something wrong?" I asked.

A dirty blond wig sat askew on her head. Only one leg, which was covered with a wrinkled cotton stocking, extended past the skirt of her housedress, and her foot was encased in a heavy black orthopedic shoe. She reeked of a sharp ammonia smell. Urine?

I remained crouched, determined to wait her out. Finally she raised her head, and said, "I don't feel good."

"Come on into the clinic. I can examine you to see what's going on."

Stella shook her head. No amount of reasoning would get her to come into the clinic or describe her problem any further. Did I really scare her that much? The ammonia odor made me think about a urinary tract infection, a common cause of general malaise in older women. I had no other plan.

"If I give you a specimen bottle will you urinate into it and bring it back to me so I can test it? Maybe you have an infection."

Later that day, Stella returned to the clinic. Still reluctant to pass over the threshold, she stopped just at the clinic door, and handed me the bottle wrapped in tissues.

I called the lab the next day. Stella did have a urinary tract infection.

She agreed to take antibiotics. Although the medication cured the infection, she still hesitated to let me examine her in the clinic.

I later found out that Stella had been a diabetic for many years. Because she didn't keep her blood sugar under control, she had developed peripheral neuropathy, a loss of sensation, in her legs and feet. She didn't realize she had stepped on a dirty tack while walking barefoot until her foot turned black. After she lost her leg, she was fitted for the prosthesis and then participated in just enough rehabilitation to be able to get around on her own.

Stella was a regular at Mattie and Mary's Friday-morning breakfasts. When she didn't show up, the women would alert me, and I would knock on Stella's door. In the security of her own apartment, she would tell me if she felt ill and allow me to examine her. She always appeared to enjoy my visit as if I were an old friend making a social call.

✶✶✶

"Wow, Ms. Bukowski was certainly something else!" Rita said after Stella had left the exam room. "She had so much wrong with her, I didn't know where to begin."

"You have to look past the labels, like old age and medical diagnosis, to see how well a person functions," I said. "It's hard to believe Stella is eighty-six and gets around as well as she does with one leg."

Rita, like me, had gone back to get her masters' degree to become a nurse practitioner after she had been a registered nurse for a number of years. She sat in the chair at my desk, Stella's chart open in front of her.

"Do you think she'll follow my suggestions on diet? I got the feeling she was just humoring me."

"You never know with Stella. You did well not to lecture to her. That for sure would have turned her off. Plus, I think you had an advantage because you spoke Polish. Stella may do what you suggest because of that."

Rita laughed.

"I'm not joking," I said. "These old folks not only need to trust, but to like their providers. Remember Stella said she didn't keep the follow-up appointment with the doctor who amputated her leg? Maybe it doesn't make sense to us, but it does to Stella."

I lifted the crumpled cloth gown from the floor and tossed it in the hamper. The covering on the exam table was clean since there was no way Stella could climb up. It was hard to examine someone sitting in a chair. Another good lesson for Rita.

The room smelled musty, like Stella. I took the can of air deodorizer from its home on top of the cabinet and sprayed.

After I reviewed and signed off on Rita's documentation, she volunteered to go down to the community room on the first floor to help with the screening. I decided to see how the luncheon upstairs was going.

The din grew louder as the elevator inched upward. When I stepped off, a couple of rambunctious three-year-olds, all arms, legs, and giggles, nearly ran me down. A teacher collared them and sent them back to the table. About a dozen children were already seated. Some of the kids picked at their food with their fingers while others jostled each other, clearly not interested in finishing their meal.

Clusters of seniors had settled at tables at the far end of the room. One of the women scowled at the children. No intergenerational mingling was evident. Where was the social, fun-loving group that had danced and laughed at Sam Levy's farewell party?

I passed a pile of little jackets and boots on the floor as I entered the next room. A line of about thirty seniors snaked up to the food table. Mattie and Mary, with perspiration on their brows and upper lips, concentrated on filling the empty plates as quickly as possible to keep the line moving.

Grudgingly, I slipped between them. Mattie scooped up the turkey, and then handed me another spoon to dish out the stuffing and gravy. Next to me, Mary tackled mashed potatoes, and Priscilla ladled out limp green beans, the sleeves of her silky blouse rolled up above her elbows.

Paper plates with single servings of yellow layer cake topped with white frosting and cut into squares were crammed on a separate table. I was glad to see the menu didn't include the usual high-fat, high-salt foods, like greens with fatback, that Mattie was fond of serving. Maybe because of the children, Mattie had toned down the selection. Certainly not because of my objections.

***

I had just started working at the Senior Clinic when I first witnessed one of these social events. There were at least eighty elders, some already eating at the tables in the larger area while others lined up at the steam table in the smaller adjacent room.

Besides Mattie, Mary, Priscilla, and Ronnie, two women who worked at the main center had come to help. The wonderful aroma from the steam table intertwined with the laughter from the staff and residents.

In spite of the festive atmosphere, I thought an opportunity had been wasted. No educational literature lying on the end of the tables to be picked up and read later by the residents. No flyers promoting the clinic. And I was almost positive that no health lecture had preceded the meal. I realized only later that Mattie had organized the luncheons in an effort to promote socialization. She witnessed much loneliness when she made home visits. Apparently Karen agreed with Mattie's suggestion to ward off isolation with communal meals since Karen had freed up funding and staff for these events.

***

The children's shrieks bounced off the walls and clouds of steam billowed into my face as I mechanically dished the food out.

"Marianna!" Laverne's voice jolted me to attention.

Through the haze, I saw her standing in front of the table with Rita at her side. The two women behind them with dropped jaws wore dark blue blouses and slacks. Laverne raised her voice to introduce the volunteer nurses while the seniors jostled around Laverne to keep their place in line.

Then Laverne stretched over the mashed potatoes, and whispered, "Thank them."

Oh, yes. I was so preoccupied with this fiasco of a luncheon that I had forgotten my manners.

"Thanks for your help with the screening," I shouted to the two agency nurses. "Why not get in line and have some lunch?"

I scooped out the food as I spoke. I wondered what the nurses, or Rita, for that matter, thought of me standing at a steam table with this cacophonous surround-sound. What was I doing here? Shouldn't I have visited the health screening instead?

Money, time, and effort had gone into the luncheon. However, the children never did sing the song they had rehearsed. They and their teachers left the community room in a shambles. The seniors ate quickly, and left.

The intergenerational love-in was a flop.

31

The Talky-Walky

"Nana is acting real weird," Doug said over the phone.

"What do you mean?"

"She's following after me saying 'Don't be afraid.' And she chased me around the dining room table."

"Oh, my goodness. What did you do?"

"I finally just darted away. I *am* faster than her."

Yes, I suppose a sixteen-year-old boy can outrun a seventy-eight-year-old woman." "Where is she now?"

"Sitting on the sofa."

"How does she look?"

"Fine. She looks like Nana. Nothing different. But she's sure talking crazy."

Doug's voice was steady. He didn't sound jarred by my mother's bizarre words and actions. My watch showed four o'clock. I could leave a little early.

"Doug, I'm coming home now. Just try to keep her calm."

"Okay," he said as if this kind of thing happened every day.

I closed the patient's chart I had been working on, and placed it on top of others piled on my desk. As I unlocked the bottom drawer to fish out my purse, my hand trembled. Years ago, when I was in my teens, Mom and I went out to lunch with Carol and her mother, and Mom mentioned she once spent time in a mental hospital. Afterward, I asked Mom why she had gone into the mental hospital.

"I never said any such thing!" she snapped.

I never asked again. Maybe I was afraid what she would tell me.

I collected my jacket from the hanger on back of the office door.

In the waiting room Rosie was talking on the phone.

"Don't forget your appointment tomorrow with Mrs. Crane at two," she told one of our patients.

At the end of the day, her lipstick was still bright red, and her black hair fell neatly onto her shoulders. "See you tomorrow," she said, and hung up.

I told Rosie I had something going on at home.

"I'll come in early tomorrow to finish the charts. Just leave them on my desk."

"Sure thing. Hope everything's okay," she said as I dashed out the door.

I jogged down the stairs. It wasn't the day to get stuck in the elevator. What was going on with Mom? She had never been a predictable person. If she did have some serious mental problem, wouldn't I have seen some evidence of it by now? Sure, she flared up at inappropriate times and had an inclination for histrionics, but she had never done anything this weird. I just hoped Doug could keep her calm until I got home.

As I drove along Chicago Avenue, my mind drifted. I saw Mom wringing her hands as she wandered about the kitchen. She took the steel knife from the drawer that her brother, my Uncle John, had used

for dressing deer he hunted and that she now used for slicing vegetables. She followed behind my unsuspecting son—raising the knife.

I slammed the brakes just in time to stop at a red light and waited
for someone to barrel into my rear bumper. When no one did, I
flipped on the radio, turning the volume up.

The eight-mile drive seemed like twenty. Finally, I pulled the car
into the garage and raced to the house, stepping over Mittens as she
flopped down doing her welcome-home wiggle on the walkway.

The kitchen door was unlocked. I dropped my purse on the bar
and threw my jacket over the stool. Tiptoeing into the living room, I
saw the top of Mom's white head jutting above the back of the sofa. To
the right, Doug rested against the door jamb with his arms crossed,
vigilant. He raised a couple of fingers in salutation without taking his
gaze off his grandmother.

Walking around to the front of the sofa, I observed Mom clothed
in her usual cotton housedress and scruffy slippers. She seemed to be
listening to something Doug and I couldn't hear.

I sat down beside her. Her farmwoman's hands were folded in her
lap. I put my hand on top of them, feeling their coolness. She turned
toward me, wild eyes snapping open. I shivered.

"How are you doing, Mom? What's happening?"

"Oh, you know," she said in a whisper. "You know what's happening."

"No, tell me," I leaned closer.

"He has a talky-walky," she said, jutting her chin toward Doug.

My fear vanished, and I almost laughed.

"He does? Why is that, do you think?"

She flung off my hand as her own hands flew off her lap, and landed
hard on her thighs. "You know!" she shouted.

My heart galloped at her sudden agitation. Keeping silent, I
watched as she slowly lost interest in her own protest. When she

clasped her hands in her lap, and settled back against the sofa cushions, my clinical persona took over.

"What's your name?" I asked her.

"Jean Polumbo," she said without hesitation.

Didn't she think it strange her daughter was asking her name?

"Who am I?" She peered at me but didn't answer.

"Who is he?" I pointed to Doug, standing calmly by the door,
dressed in jeans and a long-sleeve striped shirt.

She glared at him.

"He's got the talky-walky."

She's delirious, I decided.

"I'll be right back."

I heaved myself up from the sofa, and tugged at Doug's shirtsleeve.
He followed me into the kitchen.

We stood by the sink filled with dirty breakfast dishes—an unusual
sight, and further evidence of my mother's confused mental state. The
top of my head reached Doug's chin, yet he was still a child. A pang
of guilt surfaced as I recognized I had entrusted him to monitor this
crazy, unpredictable woman. No close grandson-grandmother relationship had existed for some time, not since Mom had begun to burst
into his room to reprimand him for its untidy state, and still he duti-
fully watched her. I gave his arm a gentle squeeze.

The kitchen was quiet. No pots bubbling on the stove, no aroma of
fresh bread baking in the oven. Normally, Mom would have started
dinner by now.

Doug waited for me to speak.

"When did this start?" I asked.

"When I got home from school. She was in the kitchen just roaming
around. Then she started to yell at me to give her the 'talky-walky.'"

"Hmm. She was just fine this morning," I said. "What is a common cause of sudden confusion in older people?" I asked myself out loud. "Usually something acute, like pneumonia or a urinary tract infection or . . ."

I was remembering something Mom had said to me yesterday.

"Or it could be a medication. Yes. That might be it. I need to check something in Nana's room."

I left Doug standing in the kitchen, and ran up the staircase to Mom's bedroom. Her arsenal of daily medications was lined up on the dresser. I searched through them. There it was: a new medication with today's date imprinted in the left corner of the label.

A muscle relaxant.

Mom had visited her doctor the day before for pain on the right side of her neck. She must have picked up the medicine this morning after the kids left for school. I opened the bottle, and spilled the pills out. She had taken two doses. I knew this particular medication commonly caused confusion in the elderly. How often I had come across patients in my practice taking a drug that caused an unwanted side effect, or a drug that had an undesirable action on another drug they were taking? This was why I needed to see all my patients' medications when they visited the clinic.

Now I wondered how long it would be before Mom's medication wore off.

I scooped the pills back into the bottle and slipped the bottle into my skirt pocket. From the phone in my bedroom I spoke with Mom's doctor. Luckily I had caught him at a quiet moment in his office. He agreed with me that her agitation and paranoia were probably due to the medication.

"The drug should be out of her system by morning," he said.

Relived, I hurried down the stairs to give Mom the once-over, then started dinner.

The following morning I woke up sooner than usual, nervous about what I would find. I had put Mom to bed early the night before after a light supper. She was not in her room. As I walked down the hall, and into the kitchen, I smelled fresh brewed coffee. She was sitting at the table reading the morning paper. As usual, she had set the table. Ernie was upstairs in the shower, and the kids were getting dressed for school.

"Good morning, Mom." She looked up from the paper.

"What are you doing up so early?" she said, her voice and behavior back to normal.

"I have to go in to finish up some work from yesterday. Remember I came home early because you weren't feeling well?" She shook her head. "You don't remember the talky-walky? You seemed to be angry with Doug because he didn't give it to you."

"I don't remember," she said flatly. She had no recollection of her abnormal behavior, and didn't seem in the least bothered by my description of what had happened the day before.

As Mom turned the pages of the newspaper, a sudden feeling of protectiveness toward her flooded over me. Even though she was unaware that she benefitted from my gerontological expertise, it pleased me to know that I had discovered the cause of her erratic behavior.

32

Save One, Lose One

Agnes Larson was one of a handful of patients Priscilla had begun visiting long before the Senior Clinic opened.

"She's eighty-eight. Seems in good health. But she's losing weight, and won't come to the clinic," Priscilla told me one morning.

"Maybe if she meets you, she'll decide to come in for an evaluation." This was the closest Priscilla had ever come to giving me a compliment.

"Sure," I said, "I'll stop in to see her."

Ms. Larson was petite, with white hair loosely piled high on her head. A knitted vest covered a cotton dress dotted with pink flowers.

"How nice to meet you," she said, and extended a bony hand for me to shake. "Have a cup of tea?" Her voice was infused with warmth.

"Thank you, yes."

I usually declined eating or drinking in patients' apartments, but then Ms. Lawson was not a patient—yet.

"I drink Earl Grey most often, and occasionally I will steep Darjeeling." Her speech was free of any definable accent.

She talked about the weather, Chicago politics, and Priscilla's "delightful visits" while she boiled water in a saucepan.

I settled into a flowered sofa, a fluffy pillow behind my back, and a china cup and saucer balanced on my knee. A faint scent of roses wafted from a glass bowl filled with dried petals centered on an end table. Ms. Larson sat in an overstuffed chair adorned with lace doilies. She lifted the teacup to her lips, her gnarled hands more steady than I'd expected, and sipped slowly. Her apartment, as tidy as she, transported me out of the dingy high-rise on the gritty west side of Chicago to a pleasant country cottage. I imagined a butler would soon appear to announce that lunch would be served. How did this woman wind up in a subsidized apartment run by the CHA?

Enjoying the ambiance, I almost forgot my mission. I took a deep breath. "Ms. Larson?"

"Call me Agnes, please."

"Agnes, as Priscilla has probably told you, she asked me to come here today because she is concerned about your weight loss."

"Oh pish-posh. I'm just eating less."

"Well, why don't you come up to our clinic anyway? Priscilla said that it's been years since you had a check-up."

I almost gasped at the instant change in her expression, her mouth a thin line in her frozen face.

"No, thank you. I want nothing to do with the medical community."

"No dice," I told Priscilla later.

"Agnes Larson doesn't want to know why she's losing weight. And she sure doesn't want to come up to the clinic."

We were in the middle of our weekly Team Conference. The door to the clinic was closed. Ingrid sat next to Priscilla while Mattie and Mary, as usual, sat in chairs closest to the door. Only Priscilla and I had brought our lunches.

"Agnes Larson, Agnes Larson," Mattie said. "I don't know who she is."

"She keeps pretty much to herself," Priscilla said, lifting a fork full of salad from a plastic container precariously perched on her lap.

"I'll give it one more try," I said before Ingrid could chime in and tell me to do everything I could to get her to register in the clinic. She always supported Priscilla.

I balled up the wax paper that had held my ham and cheese sandwich and shoved it into the paper bag. I didn't like giving orders to patients. Instead, I gave them the facts and helped them understand the trade-offs.

Later in the week I went down to Agnes's apartment. She seemed happy to see me. When she offered me tea, I declined. This visit was pure business and I plowed right in.

"I've come to encourage you to come up to our clinic."

Again, Agnes grew tense.

"What is it about the medical establishment that you object to?"

Her shoulders slumped. She walked over to the chair and slowly eased herself into the seat. She remained silent for a minute as if deciding to tell me her story.

"I wasn't married more than a few months when my husband and his mother locked me in the guest bedroom, telling me I was crazy."

I dropped down on the sofa.

"I wasn't crazy," she said emphatically. "I don't remember how long they kept me in that bedroom. But finally they took me to court, and had me committed to a mental hospital."

The afternoon sun had begun to set. The living room receded in long shadows, and Agnes's voice took on a ghostly quality.

"At first I was kept on a locked unit. After a while, I suppose the nurses thought I was no threat to anyone, so I was moved to another floor. Eventually, I was assigned to work in the laundry."

Agnes' silhouette shifted in the chair, but she continued in a mono-tone as if speaking of someone else.

"Soon I was allowed to walk on the grounds unattended. Finally, because of my good behavior, I was permitted to go to town once a week on the hospital bus."

She sat quietly for a long while. A lighter voice broke the silence.

"One day when I was in town, I just walked away. I never went back. No one ever came for me."

I waited for her to say more.

Finally she added, "I never told anyone about this."

Questions raced in my mind: How did you manage to get away? Did you take anything with you—money, clothes? And why are you telling me this?

The story sounded both plausible and outrageous. I could imagine her husband's family getting away with committing her. Once inside an institution in those days, people got lost. Perfectly sane folks could stay in a mental hospital their whole lives. Agnes didn't seem to be prone to delusions, but then I hadn't known her long.

I shook myself out of my reverie.

"Do you mind if I turn on this lamp?" I asked.

The glow of the light fell on a doleful Agnes. How horrible to have lived with this secret all these years. True or not, it was a great story.

✱✱✱

The next morning, before I had a chance to call my first patient, Mabel Fitts slipped by Rosie and zipped into the exam room. Mabel surprised me by flopping onto the chair next to my desk. Although she had encouraged others to come to the clinic, including her good friend Pearlie Banks, she had refused to register herself.

Mabel jerked up her pink sweater, exposing her breasts. "I got a lump. Here." She pointed to her left breast. "Just feel it," she said. "That's all I want you to do."

Then she took my hand, and guided it to her coffee-colored breast. "Here it is."

My fingers found what felt like a hard kernel of corn. She shook my hand away, and yanked down her sweater. "I'll come back for you to check it again." *Zoom.* She was out the door.

All this happened so fast, but I got the message. Mabel didn't want to find out if the lump might be cancerous. In the mid-eighties, we didn't talk openly about cancer. We used euphemisms like "lesion" or "lump" for "tumor," because tumor meant cancer. I didn't have time to figure out how to deal with Mabel. I took the chart resting in the bin on the door, then called my first patient.

After clinic was over, a vision of Mabel darting out of the room surfaced. She must have had some faith in me to ask me to feel the lump. Would she eventually stay long enough to hear my advice and follow it? After all, she knew I had kept her friend, Pearlie, well and out of the emergency room for all the time I had cared for her—almost a year. Pearlie weighed herself daily on a scale bought by the clinic, and adjusted her water pill by following a regime that I had taught her.

Mabel had informed me that Pearlie's daughter had persuaded Pearlie to move in with her, and within a couple of months she also reported that Pearlie had died.

I was angry with Pearlie's daughter because she took Pearlie away just when she was doing so well, took her to another provider who probably had no knowledge of geriatrics or how little things can keep an older person from hitting the skids. She hadn't bothered to ask for Pearlie's records to be forwarded. Maybe she never registered Pearlie for any health care. I'd never know, but I did know that I would miss Pearlie—and her ever-present baby-food jar spittoon.

I'd have to wait for Mabel to let me examine her more thoroughly. I didn't want her to avoid me because I insisted she needed a biopsy. After working in the clinic, I had learned that some folks would chance dying from an unknown disease rather than have a test to find out what was wrong.

Over the next few weeks, Priscilla reported Agnes Larson was becoming progressively weaker. At last Agnes agreed to come to the clinic. Her gaunt face managed a slight smile when Priscilla rolled her wheelchair into the exam room.

"Hi, Agnes. Good to see you," I said, trying to keep my face from betraying my shock.

Priscilla and I eased Agnes onto the scale.

"One hundred and three pounds," I said.

"Oh dear," Agnes said, "I used to weigh 150." Priscilla eyed me with concern as she left so I could examine Agnes.

Sometimes older people lose weight as they age, and eventually their weight plateaus. Most of the time, there is no reason for that loss. However, when I examined Agnes, I found two swellings—one in the middle of each pancake breast. Maybe what I was seeing was an abnormality of her ribs? But when I touched the masses, they felt rock hard. Oh my, what else could it be but cancer? A deep sadness came over me, and I paused a moment to compose myself before I spoke.

"Agnes, how long have you had these lumps in your breasts?"

Agnes was ready for me. Twisting her mouth into a tight line, she said, "I don't care if it's cancer. I'm not worried. I've led a full life."

At least up to then, Agnes had been able to take care of herself. If I had caught the cancer earlier, she'd probably have had a few more good years. I didn't ask why she hadn't told anyone because at this point, what difference did it make?

Priscilla wheeled Agnes back to her apartment. On her return, she stormed into the examination room.

"You should have examined her sooner," she shouted at me. "If you had caught it . . ." Her voice trailed off.

"Priscilla, Agnes didn't want anything to do with the clinic. What could I do?"

I waited for Priscilla to tell me. She had never held back criticism of my practice, but I hoped she would not bring Polly Tomaski up again.

I often thought about Polly, a jovial Polish-speaking woman who frequently popped into the clinic since her apartment was down the hall. I couldn't recall ever seeing her upset even when she was diagnosed with skin cancer on her nose. The deep surgical incision removed the cancer but left her prone to hemorrhage. She often went to the emergency room to stop the nose bleeding.

"Don't bend over," I cautioned her more than once, pantomiming the gesture. She would nod but in a couple of days, I would learn she had taken another trip to the ER.

When Priscilla told me that Polly had died, I assumed it was from a hemorrhage.

"It was a heart attack." Priscilla had heard from one of Polly's doctors.

"Heart attack, my God! She came into the clinic last week pressing her fingers into the middle of her chest," I said. "I figured she had chest pain, and thought of doing an EKG but Polly ran out of the clinic as quickly as she came in. Then she was out of my thoughts. I should have done the EKG."

"Yes, you should have," Priscilla said flatly. "Then Polly would be alive today."

Priscilla displayed a strong attachment to her patients. But what gave her the right to question my actions?

She was as judgmental over my treatment of Agnes as she had been over Polly's. What could I have done when Agnes hadn't been willing to see me? I couldn't force every older person living in the building to have a complete check-up so I could find out if she had a life-threatening disease.

A familiar feeling of insecurity appeared. I was back in nursing school. A phantom was tapping me on the shoulder whispering, "You are not cut out to be a nurse. You left that woman alone in the utility room. You failed to complete your assignment."

After Rosie had left for the day, locking the door behind her, I sat in the darkened office and continued to berate myself for causing both Polly's death and Agnes's impending one. Even as I dug up more patients in my past that may have been affected by my shortcomings, I always came back around to the woman I had left on the stretcher in the utility room.

After many minutes, I stood.

"Enough," I said aloud. "Time to move on." And I bottled up my insecurities until the next time I would be forced to acknowledge I wasn't perfect.

Mabel came back the next week, again without an appointment, asking me to feel the lump. She was happy to hear me say it didn't seem any bigger. She left quickly before I could suggest a biopsy. However, each time she zipped into my office, she stayed a little longer. Finally, she agreed to let me find a doctor who would do the biopsy.

Dr. Franklin practiced at the small community hospital a few blocks from the clinic. When I mentioned that Mabel would not be eligible for Medicare for a few months, he told me the hospital had an indigent fund that would cover her costs. Mabel had the biopsy. Not surprisingly, the result was cancer.

I drove Mabel to the hospital to have a mastectomy. That way I would be sure she showed up. I parked at the entrance. Before Mabel got out of the car, she handed me her apartment keys.

"If I don't come back," she said dryly, watching for my reaction.

By now we had a comfortable relationship, so I laughed. I knew that would put her at ease. If I took her statement seriously, she would know I was worried, too. I was worried, but I really didn't think Mabel would die from the operation—unless she died of fright.

∗∗∗

Agnes had become so short of breath that she agreed to go to the University Hospital. Tests showed she was anemic. True to form, she rejected getting a blood transfusion. Too weak to go back to her apartment, she stayed in the hospital refusing food and drink.

Before visiting her, I made a two-block pilgrimage from the hospital parking lot to Lake Michigan. The waves lapped on the beach, reminding me of the Atlantic Ocean of my childhood. Needles of wet wind stung my face. As always, the sound of the surf rejuvenated me even on a blustery afternoon. With my coat collar turned up and hands tucked into my sleeves, I walked back, ready to see Agnes.

The antiseptic smell of the hospital corridors immediately recalled the days when I wore a white uniform and scurried up and down the halls checking dressings, dispensing medicine, and answering call lights. I never knew what happened to a patient after he left the hospital, unless he died on my shift. Now, in the clinic, I was entrenched in my patients' lives.

Inside her private room, Agnes lay motionless.

"Agnes," I said as I sat on the bed beside her.

She didn't move when I touched her shoulder. I found a moisturized Q-tip on the end table and spread the gel on her parched lips.

"Agnes, it was a pleasure knowing you," I said, hoping she could hear me.

I sat in her room for a while then told her goodbye when I left.

As I passed the nurses' station, I thought it sad that the nurses that cared for Agnes every day never got to hear her story. After years of imprisonment in the mental hospital, she had established an independent life and courageously followed her own counsel.

Two days later Agnes died.

The following Monday morning, Mabel was waiting for me to change her dressing. Before she left the hospital, Dr. Franklin had told her he had cut out all the cancer. Her lymph nodes were negative.

Weeks later she continued to stop by the office just to give me a hug—her hugs validated that I could save a patient and also softened the memories that haunted me.

33

Josie and Margaret

No flowering trees signaled the onset of spring in the concrete waste-land around the massive apartment building I had worked in for the past year. Yanking open the glass door to the stark foyer, I noticed Margaret parking Josie, in her wheelchair, in front of the elevator.

When Margaret saw me, she ran to unlock the inner door before I got a chance to grab the key from my purse. Had she been waiting for me? My neck muscles tightened.

"Top of the morning to you," Margaret sang out in her Irish brogue, exposing black, broken teeth, and a wooden expression in spite of her hearty words.

I looked for the ice pick Margaret reportedly always carried. She was empty-handed, and the pockets of her cardigan sweater weren't bulging. Sometimes, it was said, she stashed the ice pick under Josie's lap blanket.

I kept my guard up with Margaret, and worried about Josie.

When she came from Ireland ten years ago, Margaret was much younger than sixty, the cut-off age to live in the senior building. She petitioned the CHA to allow her to live with her aunt, who then was in her early nineties. Margaret's attention had kept Josie out of a nursing home and gave Margaret a roof over her head.

She chose not to come to the Senior Clinic for health care so I didn't know what medication she was taking to control her paranoid-schizophrenic personality, or whether she took medicine at all. Her aggressive outbursts occurred randomly. Some of the residents in the building complained about Margaret's erratic behavior, but it never became aggressive enough to evict her. As far as I knew, she had never brandished the ice pick.

Up to a month ago, Margaret pulled Josie behind her as she rushed around going nowhere. When Josie became unsteady on her feet, Margaret put her in the wheelchair, and bundled her up as if to fend off an infiltrating enemy.

"How are you doing today?" I said as I pulled the blanket aside to see Josie's pixie face. She blinked. My neck muscles relaxed. At times I fantasized that Margaret would push Josie around in her wheelchair after Josie was dead, and none of us would catch on until Josie started to stink.

Something had to disturb Margaret more than usual for her to wait for me this early in the morning.

"Josie won't eat. I put food in her mouth, and she spits it out."

We had been around this topic before. Margaret wanted to believe Josie was just fine, thank you. Therefore, any advice I gave could be met with a disagreeable outburst.

"Have you tried to give Josie small feedings, and soft food like pudding, ice cream or Jell-O?"

Ignoring my question, Margaret fussed with Josie's blanket.

When she finished, I added, "You can't force Josie to eat if she doesn't want to."

"Glory be, she not eating enough to keep her body alive!" Margaret shrieked to the ceiling.

Just then, the elevator doors opened with a loud scraping, emitting the usual stench: urine and beer. Last Friday was the first of the month when Social Security checks were placed in the mailboxes. Many of the old-timers here cashed their checks, walked directly to the liquor store, and spent the weekend in an alcoholic stupor.

Margaret changed the focus of her frustration, pinching her nostrils with her fingers and yelling, "'Tis an insult to the good people in this building that the drunks cavort and carry on so, pissing in public places!"

Her demeanor could have been seen as an attempt at humor, but I knew better.

An elderly man stepped off the elevator and nodded his head in greeting as he maneuvered around Josie's wheelchair. Margaret propelled the chair through the doors that the man graciously held open, and both women faded into the morning fog. I suspected Margaret would wheel Josie into the clinic later that day asking again why Josie wouldn't eat.

When the clinic first opened a year before, Margaret would saunter in holding Josie's hand, pulling her along. While Margaret's stringy hair and disheveled clothes reflected an indifference to her own appearance, Josie was dressed like a treasured porcelain doll. Her deep blue eyes held a sparkle. She didn't talk but nodded her head and smiled when spoken to. Who knew how much she understood?

While Josie was still walking, Margaret would bring her into the clinic. "Can ye weigh Josie this mornin'?"

Since Margaret refused to enroll Josie in our clinic, I kept a record of their visits in a manila folder in the top desk drawer. There was a sheet for each person who, like Margaret and Josie, wandered in occasionally for a weight or blood pressure evaluation.

Josie stood on the scale. I moved the beam until it balanced at ninety pounds. Josie began to teeter. I grabbed her arm just in time to keep her from tipping over.

I looked over my notes. "Josie was ninety-two pounds when we weighed her last week," I said.

"Mother of God! She's a bag of bones. I can't get her to gain an ounce."

I didn't mind weighing Josie although Margaret never uttered a "Thank you" or asked, "Is this a good time for us to stop in?" Since Margaret was known for mood swings and bursts of anger, I didn't object to seeing Josie every so often because it gave me a chance to look for any signs of abuse.

A couple of weeks after our hallway discussion, I spotted them— Margaret pushing Josie in the wheelchair with one hand, and lugging an IV pole with the other, rushing to the back door and out to the parking lot in a obvious effort to avoid me. The bottle hanging from the pole had a milky beige color that could only be a supplemental feeding. Josie now had a tube in her stomach, a conduit to deliver nutrients to keep her alive.

Soon rumors began to circulate that Josie had died. No one knew what happened to Margaret. For months afterwards, when I walked in the neighborhood, I kept a lookout for a middle-aged, disheveled woman talking to herself in an Irish brogue.

But I never found her.

34

The Faceoff

Mom plodded in her slippers through the hall and into the kitchen, her hair loose and wild. She had gone to bed over an hour ago.

"You like to eat, but you don't like to clean up."

She stormed toward the sink.

What was she talking about? We still had company in the living room, old neighbors who had driven up from the south suburbs, and Annie.

"Don't worry about it, Ernie and I will straighten up later." I put the bottle of Merlot I was carrying down on the counter and stood in front of the sink piled with dirty dishes. We had had a glorious Easter dinner of ham with all the trimmings.

Ignoring me, she began to roll up the sleeve of her pink chenille robe.

"I'm going to do the dishes," she said.

"No, you won't. Ernie and I will do the dishes after our company leaves," I repeated.

Annie wandered in and stopped by the stove, eyeing Mom and

me with nervous concern. I wished she wasn't present to witness our confrontation. But I was also determined not to let Mom wash the dishes. The sound of water and the rattle of pans would be heard in the living room, not conducive to an after-dinner conversation with our guests. And they might presume we wanted them to leave.

Mom stood facing me with one sleeve rolled up to her elbow. I held my stance.

From my peripheral vision, I watched Annie shudder, her feet rooted to the floor.

Then I peered into Mom's angry eyes. Where did this rancor come from? An inner reserve of force gushed through me as if I had drawn a line on the floor, challenging her to step across to the sink.

Seconds expanded. The walls of the kitchen bent around Mom and me, encasing us in a war of wills.

Waiting. Waiting. She stood inches away from me, breathing heavily, yet I held my ground.

Finally, she turned, her shoulders slumping as she shuffled down the hallway.

Annie left the room with out a word.

I leaned against the counter, composing myself. I hadn't allowed her to get her way. I didn't back down as I would have done in the past.

Then, bottle of wine in hand, I all but bounced into the living room to join our friends.

***

The next morning at breakfast, rather than the usual icy silence, Mom immediately announced she planned to move into her own apartment. "You don't need me here," she said.

"Fine," I said, not giving her the apology she expected or the validation of her worth.

On the way to work, a faint tingle of anticipation stirred me. Maybe this time Mom would really move out. Without me asking her to stay, she really had no choice.

Just the thought that she would be out of our home had made me giddy. The first thing I would do after she left would be to remodel the kitchen—and get a dishwasher.

35

Dying Against the Rules

On a hot summer day, a loud knock on my office door jolted me. Before I could say "Come in," the door was flung open. A large man in army fatigues and heavy boots stood in the doorway.

"We have an appointment for two o'clock."

His voice sounded flat, but his body was tight, coiled for lunging as he glared at me. I stiffened to see him block my only exit. Rosie would be no help if I screamed. She was a hundred pounds of woman poured into a tight skirt, teetering on stiletto heels.

I skimmed the appointment sheet on the side of my desk. "William Harvey, 2:00 p.m. physical exam." I checked my watch. It was ten minutes after two. The man remained motionless in the doorway. Maybe he wasn't out to harm me. I shoved aside the chart I had been writing in.

"Sorry to keep you waiting."

He left abruptly, returning with an older image of himself in a wheelchair.

"This is my father," he said. "He was in St. Elizabeth Hospital. Just got out yesterday."

He parked the man alongside my desk and stepped back to lean against the door jamb.

The older Mr. Harvey had dull brown skin and a friendly face. The pocket of his plaid shirt held a plastic liner stuffed with pens. His swollen feet, in dress socks that poked out of pressed trousers, rested on the foot supports of the wheelchair.

Trying to ignore the presence of his son, I gazed directly at Mr. Harvey and asked, "What can I do for you?"

"I have lung cancer," he said in a surprisingly strong voice.

Oh God, I didn't expect to hear an honest, forthright answer.

"Me and my sister want him to stay here," Mr. Harvey's son interrupted. "Here in his apartment."

"Is he going to go back to the hospital for any more care?"

I needed to know this. If Mr. Harvey was not returning to the hospital for treatment, I would be the person responsible for him. I wasn't sure that was what I wanted, at least not if Mr. Harvey's son was hovering about.

"They don't want to see him no more," the son said. "They give us this here medicine, and told us he don't need no more treatments."

He snatched a plastic bag off one of the wheelchair handles and tossed the bag on my desk where it landed with a plop. I flinched.

Disregarding the rude gesture, I spilled out the medicine bottles of various sizes on my desk. I pushed the bottles about to avoid holding them since my hands trembled slightly, hoping the son didn't notice. Some were duplications; one or two probably weren't needed. I divided the pills into two stacks.

"Continue taking these," I said as I put the pills back in the plastic bag. "I'm putting an elastic band around the others. Hold off taking them for now." I would have a better grasp of Mr. Harvey's medication regime after I looked over his medical record. I put aside that thought for the moment.

I knew the drill. The hospital didn't want to be saddled with the cost of care for this fellow. They had discharged him to his family, and hoped he wouldn't come back. Maybe the son had caused some trouble, making it easy to cut Mr. Harvey loose.

More pressing was what to do with him. How would the family be able to care for him as he became weaker, needing round-the-clock care?

I looked up at the son as he stood waiting for my response. I inhaled deeply.

"Please sit down," I pointed to the chair on the other side of my desk.

"I'm fine."

He was not making this easy on me. I turned toward Mr. Harvey.

"So what apartment do you live in?"

Small talk never hurt.

"I'm in eleven-ten."

"Have you been here long?"

"Yeah, about fifteen years."

"You must have known Mr. Coleman. His apartment was on the eleventh floor, too."

His crisp "yes" signaled me I had stepped over a boundary. Mr. Coleman was not a stellar citizen. He was probably in early stages of dementia when he had walked into the waiting room asking to be enrolled in the Senior Clinic. He carried a large black trash bag full of medicine from the VA.

Thankfully, I had read him right, and brought him and his trash bag down the hall into the laundry room. I slowly dumped the bottles out on the top of the dryer. The roaches leaped out. Since I had expected this, I didn't scream. In fact, I was getting almost blasé around roaches.

I didn't see Mr. Coleman again until a few weeks later when Luther wheeled him into the clinic, water trailing behind the wheelchair.

"Got a call from the woman who lives in the apartment under Mr. Coleman's. She had water running down her walls."

Luther's shoes squished as he parked Mr. Coleman in the middle of the empty waiting room.

"He left the water running in the tub."

Mr. Coleman, with a wet undershirt and boxer shorts plastered to his body, shivered.

"Let me get a blanket," I said.

When I returned, I tucked the blanket around him.

"His apartment got an inch of water on the floor," Luther said, looking down at Mr. Coleman. "I found him just sitting on the sofa. Good thing he was able to get himself up into the wheelchair."

Inside the bathroom, Luther and I peeled off Mr. Coleman's wet underwear and slid him into a tub of warm water to ward off hypothermia, a low body temperature that could cause death if left untreated, while we waited for the paramedics.

It wasn't Mr. Coleman's dementia that made me think he didn't make a good neighbor but what Luther said about his apartment afterward.

"What a mess! Garbage everywhere. The sink and counters full of dirty dishes and rotten food."

I knew Luther saw lots of messy quarters so when he said, "It gets worse," I swallowed hard.

"He had guns on the kitchen table and pictures of naked women taped on the walls."

The first time Mattie told me she and Mary were headed to the police station to drop off a gun, I thought it a unique occurrence. Since then, they had made several trips to the police station, surrendering guns they received from the residents for reasons I didn't try to remember.

***

I pulled out a blank sheet of paper to jot down notes while I took Mr. Harvey's history. I asked him about pain, appetite, sleep, and problems walking, and was impressed with his high level of independence.

"Let me examine you, Mr. Harvey."

I worked around the wheelchair as I listened to his heart and lungs, poked at his stomach, and pressed the softness around his ankles. Nothing abnormal except the swelling in his legs and dullness in the left side of his chest, probably where the tumor was.

After I completed the exam, I sat down again. He was in pretty good shape in spite of the cancer.

"Can't find anything troubling, Mr. Harvey."

I'd found patients needed to hear something positive after I examined them or else they imagined the worst.

"You need to get the swelling down in your legs. When you get back to your apartment, keep your legs elevated. Call the clinic if you are having any problems, like pain or shortness of breath."

I turned to his son. "I'll need your father's records from the hospital. After I review them, I'll have a better idea whether I can help him or not."

Getting hospital records could take a while. Hopefully, I wouldn't see the son in the near future.

I watched them leave the clinic. Mr. Harvey's son seemed about the right age to have served in Vietnam. Did that anger come from his stint in the Army? Dealing with his father's cancer and clashing with the bureaucracy of the health care system could be inflaming his already surly disposition. I turned my head from side to side to release the stiffness in the back of my neck.

The next morning, while I was enjoying my first cup of coffee, heavy footsteps clopped into the clinic. Mr. Harvey's son appeared in the same outfit and scowl on his face as the day before. He slapped a large manila envelope on my desk.

This time I didn't flinch.

"I would've brought them yesterday, but the clinic was already closed," he said.

My mind entertained visions of what forceful behavior he must have used to get the records from the hospital so quickly.

I pulled out a thick pack of papers from the envelope. While I read, the son stood rigid at the door.

After reading, I rested my chin on my hands. In the silence, I listened to the son's breathing. What if he doesn't like what I tell him? What if he goes berserk, attacking the messenger? I had no choice but to level with him about his father's prognosis.

"Your father's cancer has spread, and the doctors think that he won't live much longer. They say there is nothing more that they can do."

I stopped and waited for the words to sink in. I reminded myself to breathe.

He sagged against the door jamb.

"Yeah, I know that," he said.

Then he staggered toward me and flopped into the chair beside my desk. With his elbows on his knees, he buried his face in his hands.

Watching his anguish, I began to relax.

"What do you expect from the clinic?"

He raised his head, and turned toward me.

"Just that he don't suffer." His voice was pleading, but anger remained in his eyes.

"Who will take care of him as he gets weaker?"

"My sister is staying with him now."

He sighed, and lowered his head back into his hands. It was then I realized I was the one with the power. I could call the shots. I could decide whether to care for Mr. Harvey at home—until he died.

∗∗∗

Hospice wasn't yet an option in the early eighties. Most patients died in the hospital. Even if the family wanted to care for their loved one in familiar surroundings, the CHA allowed family to move in only after a written appeal was made. A decision to grant the request could take weeks if not months.

Sam Levy had looked the other way when the clinic stepped in, and never insisted the rules be followed. I wouldn't have been so concerned if Corrine Fitzgerald hadn't recently come on board as the new building manager after a few temporaries. I had no idea whether or not she adhered strictly to company policy. She would have the final say over whether Mr. Harvey's daughter could stay in the apartment.

The man in the seat next to my desk, dressed inappropriately for the warm summer weather, holding his head in his hands, no longer seemed so threatening. I started to reach out and touch his shoulder, but caught myself.

"I'll take care of your father," I said instead.

Mr. Harvey's son stood up and left without a word.

Later that day, I hiked up one flight to the eleventh floor. I followed the aroma of chicken soup that seeped under the door of an apartment where a large, matronly woman with smooth cocoa skin and a sympathetic smile greeted me. "I'm Sylvia," she said.

Mr. Harvey sat in a wheelchair facing the television set. I dropped down on the sofa beside him.

"You look good today. Any pain?" I asked.

"Nope."

"Did you sleep okay last night?"

"Yep."

Without his son hovering over him, I wanted to know how he felt about staying in his own apartment as he grew more ill. It wasn't a question I felt comfortable with, but if I were going to defend his request to Ms. Fitzgerald, I had better be sure that was what he wanted.

"Mr. Harvey, tell me what you want to do if your condition worsens. Do you want to go to the hospital or stay here?"

I couldn't bring myself to say, "Stay here to die."

Mr. Harvey proved more direct than I.

"I want to die here in my own place."

I was awed by his acceptance.

Sylvia had wandered from the kitchen as Mr. Harvey and I talked, her hand over her mouth stifling a sob.

Afterward, I sat at the kitchen table across from her. Did she plan to stay with her father throughout his illness? How did she feel about seeing him get weaker and eventually die?

"The good Lord will give me the strength I'll need," she said.

I had no reason to doubt her. If there hadn't been such a strong family resemblance I would have never thought that the man with smoldering anger really was her brother.

Later that week, I knocked on the open door to Corrine Fitzgerald's office. I had met her a few weeks ago as she stood among the unpacked boxes.

She had waved a feminine wand over the space. An African violet sat on the corner of her tidy desk, pictures of rivers and mountains hung on the walls, and a floor lamp in the corner canceled the need for the fluorescent lights glaring from the ceiling.

She stood when she saw me. Her beige suit and patent leather heels made her look more like an English professor than a city employee.

"Hi, come on in," she said.

I hoped I wasn't in for a battle as we shook hands.

"Sit down. What brings you here?"

Before I brought up the Harveys, I noted an interesting book on her desk: *Counseling Skills*.

"I'm taking evening classes to become a social worker."

That's when I knew I would have her support.

I obtained a hospital bed for Mr. Harvey and placed it in the living room, leaving the bedroom for his daughter. Over the next few weeks, he became weaker, and finally bedbound. Sylvia kept him clean and free of bedsores. I visited frequently. Usually two or three relatives sat around the table. If her brother visited, I never saw him. For that I was grateful.

When I walked into the lobby after the long Fourth of July weekend, Ms. Fitzgerald was waiting outside her office.

"The police called me at home this past Sunday," she said. "It was about the Harvey family."

Who else but Mr. Harvey's son? I had been waiting for some sort of incident from him.

"A group of family and friends were having a barbecue out in back of the building," she said, frowning.

"They were drinking, and a couple of the guys fired guns into the air."

I waited for more.

"No one was hurt," she said.

I gritted my teeth, wondering what she decided to do. A resident would be tossed out on the street for that behavior, especially a family that had graciously been granted exemption from the rules.

"I declined to press charges. But I won't do so again."

Not long after the Fourth of July incident, Rosie shouted to me from the front desk to pick up the phone. It was Sylvia. Between sobs she told me that her father had stopped breathing.

I rushed out of the office and up the stairs.

The apartment door was open. I found Sylvia standing beside her father's bed, weeping into her apron. Mr. Harvey's eyes were fixed on the ceiling. I touched his cool arm, and then put my hand on his chest. No motion. I unbuttoned his pajama top, took out my stethoscope, and placed it over his heart. I slid the diaphragm of the stethoscope across his chest.

When I was sure there were no breath sounds or heartbeats, I stood up, facing Sylvia. I didn't need to speak. She stumbled toward me, her arms heavy on my shoulders. Her body shook as her warm tears soaked into my lab coat.

"I'll call the ambulance to pick up your father's body."

Before I left, I closed his eyes.

Ms. Fitzgerald had to be told that Mr. Harvey had died. As I walked toward her office, his son rushed into the lobby.

"My sister called me," he shouted. "What's happening?"

Dear God, do I tell him now, here in the hallway?

"What's happening?" he repeated.

He tromped towards me, his heavy boots clopping with each step, his voice shrill and insistent, his eyes frightened.

I had to tell him. The longer I hesitated, the angrier he would become.

"I'm so sorry," I said, then paused. "Your father is dead."

His face contorted. He raised his arm as if to hit me. Then a wail escaped from his lips. He darted past me, flung open the door to the stairwell, and raced up the stairs.

Damp with nervous perspiration, I sagged in relief.

I heard from the neighbors that Mr. Harvey's son wailed until the ambulance finally arrived—well after midnight. By morning, Mr. Harvey's family had vanished from the apartment without a trace.

36

Checking the Taverns

W e were an unlikely trio hiking through Chicago's Westside. Mary, on my left, silver-haired and pudgy, cautiously dodged cracks on the uneven sidewalk with short, quick steps. Laverne on my right, closest to the curb, strode smoothly, ignoring the pockmarked path. She was ten years younger than I, her dark skin not commonly seen in the neighborhood.

I was making a home visit. Mary came to interpret, Laverne to observe.

While Laverne completed the nursing tasks I no longer had time for, she rarely identified any service, treatment or program that would benefit a patient or the clinic—she didn't do anything other than what she was told to do. I hoped that taking her with me on this visit would instill in her some enthusiasm and self-direction.

In order to avoid the summer heat, we had left the clinic early that morning. Donna Romano, Director of Onward House, FHC's sister agency focusing on social problems, had called to tell me about the Kaminskis.

A few months earlier, a fire had damaged their house. Their new apartment was just two blocks from the Senior Clinic. When a case-worker last visited, Mrs. K looked ill, and Michael, her son, was passed out drunk on the sofa. Donna asked me to do a health assessment on Mrs. K, and to eyeball Michael.

We stopped in front of a hulking two-story house with wide steps leading up to the main door. I slipped my black nursing bag off my shoulder, dropped it onto the sidewalk, and double-checked the house number against the piece of paper in my skirt pocket.

The Kaminskis lived in the basement apartment. We marched single file through the alley alongside the house, and navigated down uneven, narrow stairs. There wasn't a doorbell to be seen, so I shoved open the heavy door. A dank draft engulfed us.

"Anybody home?" I yelled.

Having Mary and Laverne with me gave me the courage to walk toward a faint light at the end of a long passageway. We found our-selves in a living room where a diminutive woman sat on a sofa puff-ing a cigarette. The air, thick with smoke, caught in my throat. I swal-lowed hard to keep from coughing. Laverne held a tissue over her nose.

Mary seemed immune to the odor as she greeted the woman in Polish, "Dzien dobry, Pani." *Good morning, missus.*

A faded housedress hung loosely from Irene Kaminski's shoulders, and then stretched tight over a protruding belly. Her short legs dan-gled inches above the floor. A Chihuahua, his body covered with scabs, scampered back and forth across the sofa and Mrs. K's lap, yapping.

"Mary, tell her the social worker from Onward House asked us to visit."

Mrs. K was not startled. Maybe she had expected us. Since the Kaminskis didn't have a phone, Donna had given me the number for Mrs. K's daughter, Wanda. I had called Wanda a few days before, asking her to tell her mother we were planning a visit.

"I don't go there any more," Wanda had said. "My brother's so belligerent. Last time I was there, he chased me out of the house."

I heard a wet, hacking cough from the other end of the line.

"Sorry," Wanda said when she put the phone back to her mouth. "Michael's a drunk. A mean drunk. I took Mom to live with me a couple of years ago."

Wanda inhaled deeply like she was taking a drag on a cigarette.

"But she just cried and cried. She missed that no-good bastard." After another coughing spell, Wanda continued. "Now that she lives with him, he spends her Social Security check on drink. He hits her and calls her 'bitch' when he's drunk. And he's drunk most of the time."

She went on to tell me, between coughing fits, that she was sixty years old and on her second marriage. Her voice cracked as she said, "And I was just laid off from work."

I didn't get the feeling Wanda wanted her mother living with her again. Or that she would welcome any suggestion from me to stop smoking and have that cough evaluated.

✶✶✶

Mary, Laverne, and I stood in the middle of the living room, my bag heavy on my shoulder. Thankfully, we didn't have coats to take off and place somewhere. Threadbare towels covered the sofa Mrs. K sat on. Newspapers on the rug to the side of us served as a doggie bathroom— with some excrement missing the mark. From the corner of my eye, I spied a roach scampering up the wall near Laverne.

Mrs. K concentrated on lighting a new cigarette from the glowing ash of the previous one as the dog bounced over her lap. Then she reached for the folded newspaper on the cushion beside her and whacked his rump. He yelped and scampered out of sight in a ritual that probably replayed often.

Mary sat on a chrome dinette chair adjacent to the sofa, and translated both my questions and Mrs. K's responses. After Mrs. K agreed to let me examine her, Mary relinquished the chair to stand next to Laverne. Like Laverne, she folded her arms across her chest.

From my new position, I saw through the open door of the bedroom a man's body lying deathly still on a single bed. His arm hung over the edge, fingers resting on a liquor bottle.

"Ask her how her son is doing?" I said to Mary.

Mrs. K began to tear up. She didn't reply. I didn't push.

Thankfully, at the last minute before leaving the clinic, I had shoved newspapers in my nursing bag. I had gotten lazy and rarely used clean technique when making home visits. Spreading the papers on the chair's ripped vinyl seat, I placed my nursing bag on top, and carried the soap bottle and paper towels into the kitchen.

The kitchen lacked cabinets. A fluorescent tube light hung from the ceiling by a chain at either end, and threw weird shadows on dirty walls. Alert for roaches, I turned on the tap slowly before I washed my hands over the soiled dishes stacked solid in the porcelain sink.

A cloud of tobacco fumes clung to Mrs. K. Years of smoking had etched creases into her face and painted yellow stains on her fingers. She wore thick cotton hose rolled up in elastic garters just above her knees. Stained slippers clung to her feet. Blue and pink bruises streaked her arms.

"Mary, ask her how she got these bruises?"

Mary translated. I didn't understand Polish, but Mary's tone suggested that she was doing her best to be diplomatic.

Mrs. K shrugged. But why would she tell strangers that her son hit her? I would wait to revisit this issue when we visited a few more times and gained her trust.

I removed Mrs. K's slippers gingerly. When I rolled down her stockings I saw deep grooves around her thighs caused by the elastic garters. Her legs were a dusky blue. I checked for ulcerations on her skin that could be caused by poor circulation, and was surprised to find none. I tossed the stockings on the sofa, and tugged her slippers back over her swollen feet.

"Ask her to walk to the kitchen and back."

Mrs. K slid off the sofa, and waddled towards the kitchen on bowed legs. On the way back, she winced with pain.

Except for the poor circulation, and pain in her legs on walking, I found nothing terribly wrong. I suggested Mrs. K not dangle her legs over the sofa's edge but keep them elevated as much as possible, and stop wearing the tight garters. Our clinic could supply support stockings to improve circulation and ease the pain. I offered to bring a lightweight wheelchair she could use to maneuver about in the small apartment.

My final request of Mary: "Tell her smoking is not good for her circulation. She would have less pain if she quit. Not to mention that smoking is a fire hazard."

Laverne hadn't made a move since we arrived.

"Anything else you would like to add?" I asked her. She shook her head.

I guessed she was anxious to leave.

Out on the street, the sun warmed my skin and elevated my mood.

"Oh, those roaches climbing up and down the walls. And that ugly dog," Laverne said. "I didn't know where to stand with all the dog poo on the rug."

I was glad to see Laverne animated, even if it was negative.

"What should we do now, Laverne?" I asked.

I wanted to hear that while she stood those many minutes in the filthy living room with an old and possibly abused woman, a dead-drunk son, and a mangy dog, Laverne had been thinking about a plan of care to make things better. Although working at FHC was Laverne's first job out of nursing school, I hired her because she was older and had had life experience. Maybe the old rule that nurses needed to work in the hospital for at least a year before becoming a community nurse was valid after all. Age and life experience didn't appear to have given Laverne an advantage.

"What can we really do for the Kaminskis?" Laverne sounded as if we should give up on them. But then she suggested, "We could visit once in a while."

"How often? Looking for what?"

Did I sound frustrated? I worried about Laverne's increasing lack of involvement. She had started off so enthusiastic when I first hired her. Maybe it was more than losing her enthusiasm—she didn't seem to care.

Not pushing Laverne any further, I said, "How about you and Mary visit once a week? Keep tabs on her blood pressure and circulation and any indication that her son is getting more abusive."

"That poor, poor lady," Mary said as we walked back to the clinic. "To live in such a dark, cold apartment." She shook her head before she added, "And to have a drunk for a son."

"Yes, it's sad," I agreed.

Laverne walked on in silence.

One day when Laverne was off, I went with Mary to visit the Kaminskis. We found Mrs. K with a cigarette dangling from her lower lip, scrubbing clothes on a washboard in a large basin of soapy water in the middle of the kitchen. Wet socks and underwear hung from the clothesline strung across the room. The folded wheelchair rested against the refrigerator, but Mrs. K was wearing the support stockings.

One out of three!

A cough echoed from the living room. Mary and I hadn't spotted Michael in the recliner when we walked in. Laverne had told me after previous visits that Michael was either passed out in his room or wasn't home.

That moment might not happen again. I grabbed a chair, and sat beside him. He stank from a mixture of alcohol, tobacco, and blood. I wondered if he was vomiting blood. Not a good sign.

Two pictures sat on top of the silent television that I hadn't noticed. One was of an attractive, dark-haired young woman, and next to her, in a matching frame, a handsome soldier wearing a green uniform covered with medals. In all likelihood, the soldier was Michael. Was the woman his wife? Wanda had told me Michael started to drink heavily after his wife died.

I saw no similarities between the soldier in the picture and the derelict in front of me with matted hair, gray chin stubble, and scrawny legs covered with spidery blue veins jutting from boxer shorts. In his mouth, a cigarette with a long ash was hanging dangerously over his distended belly and grungy undershirt dotted with burn-holes.

Michael's rheumy eyes glared at me. With no empathy for this slovenly man, I avoided any pleasantries.

"Michael, why do you drink so much? Why do you hit your mother?"

He sniveled, squirmed, and emitted a sound almost like a howl. He started to weep.

His mother hobbled from the kitchen, soapsuds dripping down her arms. She rested a wet hand on Michael's shoulder as tears ran down her cheeks.

I heard a muted sob from behind. Don't tell me Mary was crying, too. My own throat tightened. What was I thinking? I had always prided myself on not showing frustration. But the thought of Michael beating his mother drove me to lose control. I leaned forward, and tried to muster the right mixture of authority and concern.

Ignoring Mrs. K clinging to her son's arm, I said, "Michael, your drinking is killing you. I want to admit you to the hospital where you can get treatment."

The very mention of the word *hospital* set Mrs. K off into a crying frenzy, and Michael began spewing curses. I was lucky he was too drunk to raise himself from the chair to hit me.

Soon the force of his anger left him exhausted. He dozed off. Mary patted Mrs. K's hand, speaking to her softly in Polish.

Without an intervention, I imagined possible scenarios. Varicosities in Michael's esophagus would burst as a result of his drinking. With no phone in the house, he would bleed to death before anyone could arrive to help. Or maybe he would choke on his own vomit.

Then I pictured Mrs. K unable to cope with her son's death. Her daughter wouldn't want her. Mrs. K would become sicker and sicker living in that damp basement, and eventually die.

There was another scenario I didn't want to think about. What if a fallen cigarette set off a fire? Maybe a lighted cigarette had caused the fire in their previous house?

Mary and I left Michael snoring and Mrs. K back at her washboard.

I planned to speak to Laverne about visiting twice a week.

Not long after that visit, I received a call from Donna Romano.

"Michael hasn't been seen for a couple of days," she told me. "No matter how drunk he's been, he has always managed to get home before night. His mother is beside herself with worry."

It was close to noon, and I had a craving for potato and cheese pierogies for lunch. I could search for Michael on my way to the Polish deli. I'd check the taverns. Heaven knows there were plenty in that hard-drinking, blue-collar neighborhood. I had no idea if Michael even frequented taverns. But at least I'd be doing something.

A couple of blocks from the clinic, I pulled open the door to the first tavern. The odor of beer, tobacco smoke, and old wood paneling filled the room. A TV flickered on the wall. Two men on bar stools turned around and ogled me. I stayed only long enough to see that Michael wasn't there.

The next bar was livelier, with at least five men sitting on high stools, laughing and shouting at each other, but had the same stale air, flickering TV, and no Michael. I sauntered into three more, stood at the entrance, scanned the patrons, and abruptly left.

Each time men's eyes followed me out the door.

Carrying the warm pierogies in a paper sack, I traveled a different route back to the clinic. But no Michael was slumped on a bar stool, or trudging down an alley, or lying in the gutter.

The next week Laverne and Mary were heading out of the clinic to visit Mrs. K. They stopped at the door when they heard Rosie announce: "Marianna. Call for you. Jake Kaminski."

"Who the heck is Jake Kaminski?" I said. Jake, a grandson I hadn't known existed, was on the other end of the phone.

"I went to visit Grandma the other day, and found out my dad hadn't been home for a while."

While he spoke, I tried to figure out how old he was. Maybe in his late twenties?

"I called the hospitals. Community Hospital had a John Doe brought in over the weekend. A middle-aged man with no identification on him found dead in an alley."

His voice broke as he continued.

"They took me to the morgue. It was my father. They said he bled to death."

"Oh, Jake, I'm so sorry." I felt both sadness and relief.

Mary plopped down in my desk chair, and put her head in her hands. Laverne stood rock still.

"I'm not saying I'm gonna miss him," Jake said, back in control. He told me he planned to pack up his grandmother's belongings, and take her to live with him and his family in a south Chicago suburb. "Grandma gave me the brochure you left at her place. She asked me to call, and thank you for all you did for her—and my father."

That was one ending I had never imagined. The other was the letter of resignation Laverne left on my desk a week later.

37

Friday Night Blues

Priscilla breezed into my office as I prepared the agenda for the team meeting later that day. With the warmer weather, she had discarded her woolen cardigans for floral blouses, but still wore swirly skirts and practical low-heeled shoes.

"I want to tell you about a lady I'm seeing." True to form, Priscilla didn't ask whether she was disturbing me.

"She seems tired. She could be losing weight. I want to get her up to the clinic, but she refuses. How about coming on down to her apartment and meeting her?"

I hoped this wasn't another Agnes Larson who just wanted to be left alone.

"I have time now. Let's go." I put my pen down, and pushed my chair away from the desk.

I stared at Priscilla's dark brown hair flecked with gray as she walked down the stairs ahead of me.

"Maria Avello has no family," she said over her shoulder. "She has her Social Security check sent to a disc jockey on an Italian radio station. He pays her rent, then mails her money for food—not enough to live on, but she doesn't want me to contact him."

"A disc jockey? How crazy is that?"

"He comes from the same town in Italy that she comes from," Priscilla said, as if that explained it.

She stopped on the landing in front of the exit door with the number six hand-painted on it. We entered a quiet hall. Every floor had its own character. Not only was this floor somber, it lacked any cooking odors like greens with ham hocks, or sauerkraut, or my favorite—freshly baked bread.

Priscilla knocked twice, then opened Maria's apartment door. The small woman, all in black, stopped fingering the rosary in her lap and turned to us.

"Hi, Maria," Priscilla said like it was every day we dropped in, uninvited.

This scene was getting all too common. Unlocked door. Dingy apartment, sparsely furnished. Silence. Depression.

Priscilla sat down in the chair beside Maria, taking one of Maria's hands into hers—an uncharacteristically tender gesture.

"I brought someone to see you."

Maria's mouth formed a smirk rather than a smile. It could have been because she didn't have any teeth. Priscilla introduced me, and gave me her seat.

"Maria, how are you feeling?" Maria's deeply wrinkled face remained motionless. "Do you have any pain?"

A soft, guttural "No" escaped from her lips.

She reminded me of my grandmother, right down to the braided bun on top of her head held up with bobby pins. However, my grandmother had had sons, daughters, grandchildren, and great-grandchildren in her life. I couldn't picture her alone like Maria.

When I asked her to come to the clinic for a check-up, she shook her head. I glanced up at Priscilla and shrugged. Priscilla returned my shrug. I slowly rose from the chair.

Priscilla pulled open the heavy door to the stairwell.

"I don't have a good feeling about Maria," I said. "Maybe she's depressed? Who wouldn't be in a bare apartment with only a voice on the radio for a friend?"

"Well, she has made it perfectly clear to me she doesn't want any interference with how she lives. Plus, she has been independent for the twenty years she's lived here," Priscilla said.

Case closed.

But I still wasn't convinced we shouldn't intervene. I had seen enough lonely, isolated elderly to know they were easy prey for unscrupulous individuals, like the radio deejay or "adopted" grand-daughters, and even family members.

In the past week, I had called Edna Perrino's son, Louie, to ask him for money to pay for a new truss. He cashed his mother's Social Security checks. Louie had the audacity to tell me he needed that money to pay off a new car. He left rent money and barely enough for groceries. The kind-hearted housekeeper, who was sent by the city to care for Edna, brought food from her own home.

After I got off the phone with Louie, I paid a visit to Edna and convinced her to have her checks mailed to the clinic. At least we would make sure she had control over her own funds. I hoped Louie wouldn't come after me when he found he no longer had money for his car payments.

That Friday, after everyone had left, I sat at my desk. It was time for me to go home, but images of Maria forced their way into my thoughts. I couldn't shake the fact she so reminded me of my grand-mother, the grandma who didn't want me to become a nurse.

✱✱✱

I had decided to enter nursing school with my new best friend, Gloria. Gloria's older sister was a nurse. The summer before we graduated from high school, Gloria's sister and her three friends—all nurses— sat around the kitchen table in a summer rental with a wrap-around porch just three blocks from the Atlantic Ocean in Avon, New Jersey.

Wearing fat pink rollers in their hair and light cotton wraps, they spun tales of busy hospital wards, joking with doctors, and being *in charge* on the evening shift. While listening to their stories, Gloria and I pictured ourselves in white uniforms, wearing white caps signifying we were registered nurses. No one mentioned illness, injury, or death.

I never told Gloria about the woman on the stretcher. I tried to assure myself that abandoning my assignment reflected my immaturity at the time.

All that was left was to pick out a school. We narrowed down our choice to two: a Catholic school in New Jersey and Bellevue in New York.

Gloria asked me, "How can you learn about nursing if you don't incorporate Catholic ethics and morality into the process?"

She gave more weight to the whole Catholic philosophy than I did. I figured it was because in grammar school she had been chosen to place the crown of flowers on the statue of the Virgin Mary in the May celebration.

While my parents supported my decision to go to nursing school, Grandma, my father's mother, didn't think it was a good idea. I visited her in her second-floor apartment to tell her my news.

"Mar-yee-anna." My name somersaulted off her tongue. "Why you wanna be a nurse? Huh?" Grandma yelled at me in her singsong voice as if I was on the other side of the room rather than right in front of her at the kitchen table.

"Hey, whana you do? You cleana da bedpans? Huh?" She came close, garlic breath warming my face as her waving hand grazed my ear. "Thata no gooda work. No gooda." Her braided bun, loosely fastened by hairpins, wobbled as she shook her head.

Her feet, with stockings rolled down around her ankles, planted themselves firmly by my chair. The pizza she made just for me, her first granddaughter, lay warm and fragrant on the Blue Willow plate in her hand. She slid the plate in front of me.

Grandma knew as well as I that in the 1950s there were few job choices, much less careers for a woman. Those in her Italian neighborhood lived in multifamily clapboard houses. They cooked the meals, raised the children, and played a supporting role to their husbands.

So Grandma expected me, too, to get married after I graduated from high school, then start making babies.

Maybe she couldn't speak English well, but she grabbed my attention. I tried to tell her why I wanted to be a nurse, but I couldn't think of a reason that would make sense even to me, much less to this opinionated old lady.

The sound of thick tomato sauce bubbling on the stove filled the silence as she waited for my answer. I could have said: I like the uniforms, Grandma. Especially the white cap with wings that will sit low on the back of my head. As a nurse, I can always get a job, Grandma. And if I quit work to have kids, I'll be better able to care for my family with all the stuff I'll learn in nursing school. And, Grandma, I picked out a Catholic school.

Instead, between bites of the pizza, I mumbled some vague remark that I knew she would not understand any more than I did, such as "nursing is a worthy profession." She gazed at me as if trying to digest what I told her. After wiping her gnarled hands on her apron, she turned and padded back to the stove.

In September 1959, Gloria and I entered St. Peter's School of Nursing in New Brunswick, New Jersey. Besides being a Catholic school, it was closest to the Jersey Shore where we had spent past summers in pursuit of sun, sand, and boys.

The deed being done, Grandma no longer badgered me.

★★★

I knocked on the door before slowly opening it. Maria sat at the table just as I last saw her, but this time she was holding a can of tuna fish. Ignoring me, she dipped her crooked fingers into the tin, carefully avoiding the sharp edges that bent over the sides. She picked up pieces of the pink flesh and shoved them into her mouth. Droplets of olive oil stuck to her chin hairs and dripped off her fingers. Her bottom jaw rotated as she gummed the fish.

"Good afternoon," I said.

Her dull eyes scanned me like an unwelcome interference.

On instinct, I walked over to the refrigerator and pulled open the door. White glare from the vacant shelves leaped out. I peeked into the cupboards and found a loaf of moldy bread and a jar of black olives.

So the disc jockey gives her money for food. Right, Priscilla.

I couldn't leave Maria in the apartment over the weekend without anything to eat. One option was to go to the grocery store myself. As I mulled that over, I noted her heavy breathing and pale skin. I regretted not bringing the blood pressure machine, thermometer, and stethoscope with me.

What choice did I have but to take her up to the clinic and evaluate her? If she needed to be admitted to the hospital, at least I would have a phone. I sat down next to Maria.

"Maria, I don't think you should be alone in your apartment. You have no food. I'm worried about you."

She ignored me as her fingers probed the bottom of the empty can.

"I want you to come to the clinic with me where I can take your blood pressure and listen to your heart. Okay?"

Maria made smacking sounds as she licked her fingers.

Damn it. What was I waiting for?

Standing up, I pried the can from Maria's grip, and dropped it in the sink. I snatched a dishtowel from the counter and wiped her oily chin and fingers. Then I dragged her walker over, and positioned it in front of her.

"Stand up, Maria." She grabbed the handles, and lifted herself up with a grunt. Her body shook with the effort. Her breathing quickened.

"No, this won't do at all." I eased her back down into the chair.

"Now what should we do?" Her strident breathing answered me. I would have to carry her.

"Heave, ho, Maria. I'm taking you upstairs to the clinic."

I slid my arms under her shoulders, bent my knees, and lifted her to her feet. Her head bumped against my chest. I bent low, looped her arm behind my neck, and hoisted her over my shoulder like a sack of clothes—dirty clothes with a faint infusion of tuna fish. She didn't cry out or struggle.

Maria was surprisingly light as she bobbed on my shoulder. No one popped his head out of an apartment to see me hauling her down the hallway. The elevator came quickly. Thankfully, it was vacant.

Inside the clinic, I settled Maria in the chair beside my desk and took her blood pressure, pulse, and temperature. She had a slight fever. Her blood pressure was low, and her heart thundered rapidly. I filled a glass with water, and handed it to her. She needed both hands to drink. Water dribbled from the sides of her mouth. My best guess was that she was malnourished, dehydrated, and anemic.

"Maria, you are going to the hospital!" I told her, and to my surprise, she didn't protest.

I phoned the ambulance service, and then the Emergency Room, and told the admitting nurse all I knew: Maria's name, address, and what I thought was wrong with her.

Friday was the worst day to deal with a patient crisis. I had spent many a Friday night sitting in the clinic, or in a resident's apartment, waiting for an ambulance. The fights, accidents, and shootings that erupted on Fridays—payday in Chicago—kept the ambulances busy. I hoped I wouldn't have to wait hours before the paramedics showed up.

I called home. Mom would feed the kids before they ran out to their teenage activities. At least my tardiness wouldn't affect them. Ernie would wait to have dinner with me.

After our argument, Mom and I had settled into a polite but cool relationship. Just as I had hoped, she didn't renege on her choice to move—she couldn't admit she had made a mistake. She found a one-bedroom apartment that she asked me to look at with her. Her Social Security check wouldn't cover the rent, but rather than suggest that she remain with us, I put her on the waiting list for an apartment in a senior building on the other side of town that charged rent based on a sliding scale. Mom could do her own shopping and cooking, and with other older folks in the building, I hoped she would make friends and socialize.

Unfortunately, it didn't have a clinic on the premises. But then I knew of only one clinic housed in a senior building—ours.

Although I knew she would regret her obstinate stance eventually, her departure promised to lift the storm clouds that had hung over me and my family for far too long. I remained anxious until her bedroom was vacant.

As I thought of Mom's departure, Delilah showed up in the waiting room with Ms. Henry in a wheelchair. Calvin was curled up on her lap.

Delilah said, "We're happy you're still here. We wanted to say goodbye."

"I'm goin' live with Delilah," Ms. Henry said, with the widest of smiles.

Delilah added, "We're gonna be a family."

I wished them well. However, my detached professional self thought Delilah might be taking on more than she could handle. As Ms. Henry grew older and more dependent, Delilah would have to navigate the health care system to keep Ms. Henry from becoming a burden. The cost in time, money, and effort could prove disastrous. But then Delilah wanted to have whatever precious time she could with Ms. Henry, regardless of the cost and effort. She seemed to be a better person than I, who eagerly anticipated my own mother's moving out of my house.

To divert myself from these thoughts, I decided to clean the top drawer of my desk. Out came pencils, pens, rubber bands, two tubes of lipstick, a comb, an assortment of take-out menus, and an array of business cards from drug representatives who visited the clinic leaving samples and educational materials.

A siren blared in the distance. I went to the window, and watched an ambulance pull up to the curb.

"The ambulance is here," I said to Maria, as I swept the items on my desk back into the drawer.

Minutes after I buzzed them into the building, the elevator door opened, and two paramedics rushed into the clinic. Luck was with me: it had been only a thirty-minute wait.

After a quick assessment, the men lifted a docile Maria onto the stretcher and neatly tucked her in. I locked the clinic and followed them out of the building, relieved she would be admitted to the hospital, not fading away in her apartment over the weekend.

It was well past rush hour. I decided to drive a few blocks out of my way to avoid Chicago Avenue, where "smash and grab" increased with the evening shadows.

I called the hospital as soon as I arrived at the clinic on Monday morning. The nurse told me that Maria had received multiple blood transfusions and was doing well. "The doctors had never seen such a low hemoglobin. She got to the hospital just in time."

Maybe I didn't save Maria's life by busting into her apartment on Friday and shipping her off to the hospital. If I hadn't taken over, what condition would she be in on Monday? I'd never know.

Maria's physical state was stable, but her loneliness would be harder to treat. She probably would be shipped to a nursing home, and her Social Security check rerouted to the home. The disc jockey would miss Maria's money, but would he miss Maria? Visit her? I hoped I had pegged him wrong, but truthfully, I figured he was just out for himself, like Louie Perrino.

38

Playing Sheriff

"**P**romise me that you won't let them Church People get my money." I was ushering Mr. Brown out of the exam room when he unexpectedly touched my arm.

I stopped and turned to face him.

"Who are these Church People, Mr. Brown? What do they want with you?"

Mr. Brown, a courteous gentleman, had been one of the first patients to see me regularly. At seventy, he had had minor health issues until he developed a heart block and had a pacemaker implanted. Without a wife or children, he often expressed fear of going to a nursing home. But I had never heard him mention Church People. His worried expression and abrupt outburst flustered me.

"They have a church on Chestnut Street. Some of the folks here go to their church. But I think they're a bad bunch of people." Anxiety spiked his words. "They come and sit in my apartment and pray. I don't want them in my place. I tell them so. But they still come around."

I wanted to ask more questions, but Rosie appeared with my next patient following behind.

"Don't let them get me. They're evil," Mr. Brown whispered as he made for the door.

The next morning, prior to the clinic's opening, Mattie, Mary, and I sat in the waiting area sipping coffee. Haze outside the casement windows predicted another sultry day.

"Stella Bukowski is moving out of her apartment. I don't know what she's getting herself into," Mattie said. "She told Mary that she'll have a room in someone's house. They're goin' take care of her for the rest of her life."

"That sounds strange," I said. "I know Stella has no family. I hope nobody's taking advantage of her."

"It's those Church People," Mary said, frowning. "They're visiting the residents, trying to get them to join their church."

"So, who are these Church People?"

"Well, me and Mary talked to two women a bit ago," Mattie said. "They were waitin' on the elevator. They dressed like nuns—in black dresses and veils—and called themselves Sister Elvira and Sister Clara." Mattie sipped her coffee, then rested the cup behind her chair on the windowsill for lack of tables in the waiting room. "They said they were inviting folks to come to their church."

"When Mattie asked her who they were visiting, Sister Elvira said that she didn't need to tell us," Mary added.

Mattie smirked, "Uppity lady." Mattie was quick to criticize those she thought put her down or acted haughty.

"Yeah," I said, "Or maybe she thought she shouldn't share confidential information." Then I made a connection that disturbed me. "I wonder if the women are the same Church People Mr. Brown told me about yesterday?"

I repeated my conversation with Mr. Brown. "How about stopping to see him from time to time?" I said. "Who knows, maybe they will invite him to move with them, too. He has no family, either."

I slipped on my lab coat. "I'll drop in on Stella later today."

Before I left for the weekend, I knocked on Stella's door, and shouted, "It's me. Marianna."

A wobbly voice called out, "Door's open."

"Hi," I said to the chunky woman relaxing in a recliner, knitting, with one leg visible on the footrest and the artificial leg propped up against the side of the chair.

I stepped into the humid room. "What are you knitting?" I asked.

"A crib blanket for the unwed mothers at St. Boniface's," she said, lifting a blue blanket off her lap.

Stella wore her curly wig askew on her head as usual. In the winter, the wig kept her head warm. But it wasn't winter. It was the middle of summer, and it felt like the tropics in her apartment.

In general, older people don't feel high temperatures, which makes them more susceptible to heat stroke. Only a handful of the residents had window air conditioners. A few more had table fans, most often bought by children who then argued hopelessly with their parents to turn the fans on.

"At least put the fan on," I said. Mattie had found a second-hand oscillating fan for Stella that sat motionless on top of the TV. I flipped it on. Stella knew better than to protest.

"Did ya hear I was moving?" she asked.

"Well, that's why I'm here," I said as I took off my lab coat. I pulled over a paisley-covered footstool, and bent low to sit on it. Careful not to spill the contents of my overstuffed pockets, I folded my lab coat and placed in on my lap.

Stella rambled on about Sister Elvira and Sister Clara.

"My, they're lovely ladies. They got a big house. I'll have my own bedroom. We'll eat all our meals together."

"What do you give them in return, Stella?"

"My Social Security check. That will pay for everything."

This didn't sound too kosher. "Have you seen the place where you'll be staying?"

"No, but they said it's really nice."

She sounded like a little girl who believed Santa would bring her a pony. It made no sense to try to convince her that this wasn't a good idea, at least until I learned more about the arrangements.

"Keep the fan on," I said before I left.

As I pulled the unlocked door behind me, I thought of my mother living in her own apartment for the last three months. She was one of the lucky ones because she had me to keep an eye on her.

Mom's move did not start out smoothly. Initially, she called me daily with vague complaints and requests. Once she asked that I stop by to close her ironing board.

"Mom, knock on your next-door-neighbor's door or go down to the office."

Mom's dependence on me dwindled when she found a friend, Pearl—a woman much younger than she who had had a stroke, and walked unsteadily with a cane. She held on to Mom for balance. Her vision was better than my mother's so they compensated for each other's handicaps. Yet Mom was suspicious of her. "You know," she told me when I last visited, "I think Pearl didn't really have a stroke. She just wants sympathy."

I didn't comment since I knew I wouldn't convince her other-wise. I also knew that when I left her building, I would leave her paranoia and anger behind. The novelty of coming home without finding Mom working in the kitchen hadn't worn off before Ernie and I signed a contract with Sears to install a dishwasher and replace our worn kitchen cabinets. The renovation brightened the room, and without Mom living under my roof, my spirit had also brightened.

***

I forgot all about the Church People until the following Tuesday when Rosie called me on the intercom. I was with one patient in the exam room, and had two more waiting to be seen.

"Luther's out here. He needs to speak with you."

I always made time for Luther. He stood in the middle of the waiting room mopping the sweat off his face with a large handkerchief.

"Miz Crane, can I talk with you?"

The lively conversation between the women abruptly stopped.

"Come on in here, Luther."

I led him into the bathroom and closed the door behind us.

"We had a complaint about a rotten smell from Stella Bukowski's apartment. Ms. Fitzgerald sent me up to check on her." The words rushed from his mouth.

"Sit, Luther."

I lowered the lid on the toilet. Luther sat down and wiped his face again. This time I noticed his hands were shaking. He took a couple of deep breaths. I braced myself for what was coming.

Luther, a veteran of high-rise horrors, told me he had found Stella slumped dead in her recliner. Because of the heat, her body had decomposed quickly.

Had Stella died from a heart attack or low blood sugar? I pictured her as I left her with the baby blanket across her lap, and her wig sitting on her head, both elevating her body heat. Maybe the fan hadn't been enough to keep her cool. Should I have insisted that she take off her wig and stop knitting? Would that have made a difference?

Where were those Church People when they could've been helpful? I wondered if Stella's death might have been a blessing. What fresh horror might have awaited her in a home run by the Church People?

✶✶✶

Later that week, Mattie and Mary scurried into the clinic. I could hear them pant as they tromped up to my desk.

"You need to come with us right away," Mattie said.

She stood so close to me I could smell the peppermint Tic Tac on her breath and sense her determination. I closed the chart I was working on and turned in my chair.

"The Church People are with Mr. Brown. They won't let us in. A young man came to the door with his fly open. I couldn't see Mr. Brown in the apartment. Come on."

How could I refuse? Finally, a chance to see what these Church People were up to.

"Give me a minute to put on my lab coat. I'll appear more official."

"It's faster to take the stairs," Mattie said as the three of us trekked out of the clinic to save a man imprisoned in his own apartment. No one talked, as if talking would delay reaching our destination.

As I followed the women down the stairs, I had to acknowledge that the clinic's location in the senior high-rise proved beneficial. Showing up unannounced had its merits.

Mr. Brown's door was ajar. I shoved it open. The first thing that caught my eye was a thin, dark-skinned young man standing across the room, reading aloud from a Bible. To his left, Mr. Brown leaned against the wall with the startled look of a trapped animal.

The window air conditioner buzzed in the background. A woman sat on the sofa in a long black dress trimmed with white ruffles at the neck and sleeves, and a short black veil on her head. Her eyebrows leapt with surprise at seeing three women barge into the apartment. Quickly she turned her attention to the kitchen table to my left where another woman, dressed in similar garb, was absorbed with papers set out in front of her, unaware of our arrival.

The woman at the table must have felt her friend staring at her, or noticed the young man had stopped reading, or else she felt our presence. She turned toward me. "What are you doing here?" she said in a high-pitched voice.

Before I could ask her, in turn, what she and her two friends were doing there, Mattie broke in, introducing me as if I were nobility gracing my subjects with my presence.

"This is Marianna Crane, our nurse practitioner, who runs the Senior Clinic." She gestured to the lady at the table. "This is Sister Elvira," and turning to the woman seated on the sofa, "This is Sister Clara."

Mattie thought my title and position would intimidate the women. I hoped she was right.

Sister Elvira straightened herself in the chair and said, "We came to visit Mr. Brown to spread the word of our Lord. Mr. Brown has told us he would like to be a member of our church."

Sister Elvira nodded toward the young man. "This here is William."

William closed his Bible, and smiled shyly. As he moved back a couple of steps, I could see his white broadcloth shirt poking out of the zipper of his black slacks. It seemed unintentional. He was just a teenager.

Elvira continued speaking of their church, and how happy Mr. Brown was to be part of their "family." The last thing I wanted to do was engage in small talk. Ignoring Elvira, I moved toward the corner where Mr. Brown huddled.

"How are you today, Mr. Brown?" His eyes darted back and forth. I tried to move into his line of vision but he didn't take me in. "Do you recognize me? What's my name?" Nothing. "Where are you?" No answer.

I stepped closer and smelled urine. His trousers were wet. His trembling hands hung at his side. I grasped his arm, and led him to the sofa. His walked stiffly like his joints were rusted, and needed oiling. Not taking the time to look for a towel to place underneath him to protect the sofa from his damp pants, I slowly eased him down. He sat as if in a trance.

I plunked myself beside him, taking in his symptoms: confusion, tremors, and difficulty walking. I needed to get him into the hospital. He had had an abrupt change in mental status—a diagnosis guaranteed to get him admitted and evaluated.

The intrusion of the Church People angered me. Didn't Mr. Brown tell me he didn't want to join their church? There was no reason they should remain. I rose from the sofa.

"I'm going to call for an ambulance," I announced. "You all need to leave."

Sister Elvira's body jerked forward but she stayed seated. What if she refused? I couldn't let her ignore my request.

"You need to leave," I repeated, trying to keep my voice steady.

Sister Clara and the boy focused on Sister Elvira. My body tensed. I waited for her to make a move. She shuffled the papers on the table as if deciding how to proceed. Finally, she pushed back the chair with a scraping noise and stood, scooping up the papers along with a set of keys.

"Are those Mr. Brown's keys?" Mary asked.

I was grateful for Mary's sharp observation. Sister Elvira didn't answer. She clutched the keys tightly as if defying anyone to take them away.

In spite of the air conditioning, nervous sweat moistened my skin. I sidled up to Sister Elvira, inhaling an onion smell from her body. She was a head taller than I, and outweighed me by at least fifty pounds.

"Give me the keys." I was surprised my hand was steady as I reached out.

Was she going to question my authority? She clenched her lips. Maybe she sensed my anger, which began to bolster my determination to kick her and her allies out. It seemed forever before Sister Elvira dropped the keys into my outstretched palm, abruptly turned, and marched out the door. Sister Clara and William trailed after her.

Mattie slammed the door behind them.

The women, laughing and gasping, rehashed the showdown— Mary holding her belly and Mattie drying the tears from her eyes.

"We were the posse rounding up the bad guys, and Marianna was the sheriff!" Mattie gave a whoop.

"And when she asked for keys, oh my, you should have seen the look on Sister's Elvira's face," Mary howled.

As I laughed along with the women, the tension in my muscles slowly melted away. Their joy in watching the Church People file out of Mr. Brown's apartment was infectious. A warm feeling of camaraderie swept over me.

As Mattie and Mary washed and dressed Mr. Brown in clean clothing, I called the hospital to admit him and then sent for the ambulance. The women left to retell the story to Rosie and Priscilla and, I imagined, eventually to the staff in the main center. I didn't share Mattie and Mary's optimism that we had run the bad guys out of town. The Church People would probably shy away from the CHA building for a while. There were plenty of frail old folks in the neighborhood to keep them busy. They would be back, or others like them. I would be on the lookout.

I flopped onto the sofa next to a dozing Mr. Brown. The aroma of Lifebuoy soap drifted toward me. With his head tilted back and his mouth agape, he snored softly, peacefully in his innocence.

He didn't know he was being admitted to the hospital. He didn't know that the acute kidney failure would be resolved and that he would retain his cognitive functioning. He didn't know that the docs would discover he had Parkinson's disease and thought it best that he didn't live alone. He didn't know that I would find a nursing home where he would befriend a man his own age who liked to play gin rummy, too. He didn't know that I would work with the nursing home social worker to protect his bank account, preventing the Church People from accessing his money. He didn't know how good I felt doing all this for him, and later for my other patients who needed more than someone just listening to their hearts and lungs.

The ambulance arrived and whisked Mr. Brown away.

I shut off the air conditioner, locked Mr. Brown's door behind me, pocketed his keys, and walked back up the stairs to the clinic where my patients were waiting.

Acknowledgements

Thanks to:

Brooke Warner and Lauren Wise at She Writes Press for bringing this book into the world.

Members of my special writing family, Elyse Crystall, Carol Dorsey, Betsy Emerson, Linda Jay*, Michele Murdock, and Libby Plunkett, who listened to the many drafts of my stories and offered support and merciless critiques.

Ceil Cleveland who offered early critical encouragement.

Pam Haley*, Mary McKinstry, Mary Kulokowski, and Bernie Tadder who clarified my recollection of the Senior Clinic.

Marilyn Fast, the best writing buddy one could hope to have, for her endless edits.

Betty Douglas whose love of gerontology inspired me.

Carol Carberry who shared my childhood experiences and validated my memories.

Donna Ramer*, nurse practitioner, who corroborated my recall of nursing skills and knowledge from 30 years ago. I am saddened that she is not here to read the completed book.

Carol Henderson, who over the years helped me grow as a writer and offered boundless encouragement.

Lois Roelofs, fellow nurse, fellow writer, and fellow traveler, who offered on-target counsel whenever needed.

My family, Doug, Jeannine, Tim, and Serena who were a positive presence in my writing life.

My husband, Ernie, whose role expanded from supportive husband to proofreader, editor, and creative collaborator.

*Deceased

About the Author

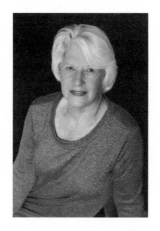

Marianna Crane became one of the first gerontological nurse practitioners in the early 1980s. A nurse for over forty years, she has worked in hospitals, clinics, home care, and hospice settings. She writes to educate the public about what nurses really do. Her work has appeared in *The New York Times, The Eno River Literary Journal, Examined Life Journal, Hospital Drive, Stories That Need to be Told: A Tulip Tree Anthology,* and *Pulse: Voices from the Heart of Medicine.* She lives with her husband in Raleigh, North Carolina.

SELECTED TITLES FROM SHE WRITES PRESS

She Writes Press is an independent publishing company founded to serve women writers everywhere. Visit us at www.shewritespress.com.

Nightingale Tales: Stories from My Life as a Nurse
by Lynn Dow, RN. $16.95, 978-1-63152-276-5
In the 1950s, nurses served as handmaidens to the physician; by the start of the new millennium, they had become admired independent practitioners. These stories, at turns humorous and compassionate, are a peek into that transition, as told by a nurse who lived it.

Catching Homelessness: A Nurse's Story of Falling Through the Safety Net
by Josephine Ensign. $16.95, 978-1-63152-117-1
The compelling true story of a nurse's work with—and young adult passage through—homelessness.

Green Nails and Other Acts of Rebellion: Life After Loss
by Elaine Soloway. $16.95, 978-1-63152-919-1
An honest, often humorous account of the joys and pains of caregiving for a loved one with a debilitating illness.

Operatic Divas and Naked Irishmen: An Innkeeper's Tale
by Nancy R. Hinchliff. $16.95, 978-1-63152-194-2
At sixty four, divorced, retired, and with no prior business experience and little start-up money, Nancy Hinchliff impulsively moves to a new city where she knows only one person, buys a 125-year-old historic mansion, and turns it into a bed and breakfast.

Role Reversal: How to Take Care of Yourself and Your Aging Parents
by Iris Waichler. $16.95, 978-1-63152-091-4
A comprehensive guide for the 45 million people currently taking care of family members who need assistance because of health-related problems.

From Sun to Sun: A Hospice Nurse's Reflection on the Art of Dying
by Nina Angela McKissock. $16.95, 978-1-63152-808-8
Weary from the fear people have of talking about the process of dying and death, a highly experienced registered nurse takes the reader into the world of twenty-one of her beloved patients as they prepare to leave this earth.